Vascular Techn

A REVIEW FOR THE REGISTRY EXAM

Vascular Technology Review

A REVIEW FOR THE VASCULAR TECHNOLOGY EXAM

2015

Donald P. Ridgway, RVT
Grossmont College and Grossmont Hospital
El Cajon, California
Editor

Barton A. Bean, RVT
BBI Vascular Laboratories
Anaheim, California
Editor Emeritus

Cindy A. Owen, RT, RDMS, RVT
Memphis Health Center
Memphis, Tennessee
Special Contributor

D. E. Strandness, Jr., MD
University of Washington
Seattle, Washington
Editor in Chief

For my mother,
Jeanne F. Ridgway,
who is largely responsible
for my growing up to be a book junkie.
—DR

Davies Publishing, Inc.
32 South Raymond Avenue
Pasadena, California 91105-1935
Phone 626-792-3046
Facsimile 626-792-5308
e-mail info@daviespublishing.com
www.daviespublishing.com

Printed and bound in the United States of America

Library of Congress Cataloging-in-Publication Data

Vascular technology review : a review for the vascular technology exam, 2001-2002 / Donald P. Ridgway, editor ; Barton A. Bean, editor emeritus; Cindy A. Owen, special contributor ; D.E. Strandness, editor in chief.-- 4th edition.
p. cm.
Previous ed. published with title: Appleton Davies, Inc. vascular technology review.
Includes bibliographical references.
ISBN 0-941022-19-6
1. Angiography--Examinations, questions, etc. 2. Blood-vessels--Ultrasonic imaging--Examinations, questions, etc. I. Ridgway, Donald P., 1948- . II. Bean, Barton A. III. Owen, Cindy. IV. Strandness, D. E. (Donald Eugene), 1928- . V. Appleton Davies, Inc. vascular technology review
RC691.6.A53 A67 2001
616.1'30754'076--dc21
2001047133

ISBN 0-941022-19-6

Contributors

Cindy A. Owen, RT, RDMS, RVT

Donald P. Ridgway, RVT

D. E. Strandness, Jr., MD

Barton A. Bean, RVT*

John B. Bennett, III, PhD

Donna E. Cox, RN, RVT*

Colleen Douville, BA, RVT

Andrew Hayes, PA-C, RVT

Margaret Johnson, RVT

Ruth Kalmer-Holmes, RN, RVT

Keith Mauney, RN*

Robert S. McGrath, RN, BSN, RVT

Cynthia Ramirez, RVT

Lars Shaw, BS, RVT

*Editors emeritus.

Preface to the Fourth Edition

WELL, HERE IT IS AT LAST, an update of Barton Bean's *Vascular Technology Review*, and it has been quite a journey. For years I have been using *Vascular Technology Review* as a text in the latter portion of the vascular technology program at Grossmont College, and I was glad to help refurbish it for the millennium. But that rascal Barton sure knew what he was doing when he said I could go ahead and work on it. Now I deserve a vacation.

Like previous editions, this edition of *Vascular Technology Review* is designed as an adjunct to your regular study and as a method to help you determine your strengths and weaknesses so that you can study more effectively. *Vascular Technology Review* covers everything on the current ARDMS exam content outline.

The new fourth edition has been thoroughly revised, updated, and expanded. While it retains the prodigious strengths and famous spirit of the first three editions (including occasionally tricky and very registry-like questions), it has changed in many other respects:

- It has been thoroughly reorganized to cover and follow the current ARDMS exam outline.

- It now focuses exclusively on the vascular technology specialty exam to ensure thorough coverage of even the smallest subtopic on the exam.

- It contains hundreds of new questions, many of which are image-based or otherwise illustrated.

- A *Hall of Images* has been added to give you even more practice with duplex images, pressures and waveforms, color flow images, and angiograms.

- Existing questions have been revised, updated, or reformulated.

- Explanations have been fortified and conveniently referenced for fact-checking or further study.

- Each section is keyed to the ARDMS exam outline so that you always know where you are, what you are studying, and how it applies to your preparation.

- A bibliography appears at the end of the book, as does the exam outline and contact information for the ARDMS.

Finally, this new edition of *Vascular Technology Review* has been approved for 12 hours of continuing medical education (CME) credit by the Society of Diagnostic Medical Sonography. The CME application appears toward the end of the book in Part X.

Effectively used, this simulated examination will help you experience the atmosphere of the exam. Current ARDMS standards call for approximately 170 multiple-choice questions to be answered during a three-hour period. That means that you will have about 1 minute per question. Timing your practice sessions according to the number of questions you need to finish will help you prepare for the experience of taking this exam. It also helps to ensure that your mock-exam score accurately reflects your strengths and weaknesses so that you study more efficiently and with greater purpose in the limited time you can devote to preparation. Because the content of this Q&A review is formatted and weighted according to the registry's outline of topics and subtopics, you can readily identify those areas on which you should concentrate.

A few of the questions depart from the usual registry format. I've left them in because they deal with useful information in a different way. And there will be some repeat questions on the same issues to reinforce key concepts and principles. These aberrations aside, the questions are designed to closely reflect what you will encounter in the registry exam. As in the exam, some questions are easier, some more difficult or obscure.

We strongly recommended that you review test-taking strategies by reading *Coping with the Exam* in this book and perhaps also by referring to one of the many books written on taking multiple-choice examinations such as the SAT, MCAT, GRE, and LSAT. The principles are the same. Such guides can increase your confidence and your performance by explaining how standardized multiple-choice exams are designed and describing practical strategies for taking and passing these tests.

LET ME JUST TELL YOU, it absolutely is *not* easy to write good multiple-choice questions. You should keep that in mind when you take the registry exam. Those ARDMS folks put a lot of effort into sorting out questions in easier versus more difficult categories, keeping the distribution even over many topics, and generally making the test challenging but not vicious or—worse—incomprehensible.

Inevitably there will be the occasional question on the actual exam that isn't quite clear or has ambiguous answers, and you will wish you could argue with the ARDMS about it. But you can't; that's the nature of this kind of exam. It is for gatekeeping, not teacherly feedback to help you to learn. The point is to do the best you can on those troublesome questions, and nail the rest. You do not need 100% correct to pass, right? Generally, you must answer between 65% and 75% of the questions correctly in order to pass, depending on the difficulty of the particular exam. And some of the questions you will be asked— approximately 15%, in fact—are trial questions that do not count. These questions, which are not identified for you, are being evaluated for use in future tests. So you can let them have a few and not get upset.

I myself have had occasion to take the vascular registry exam twice: I originally passed it in 1985, and then I received permission to take it again six years later (not officially scored), as a personal challenge and to make certain I was teaching in the mainstream of what we need to know to be smart technologists and sonographers. Both times I felt that the exam was fair and reasonable and that I would not want someone working on me who could not pass it.

We cannot guarantee that this book gives you exactly the questions you will encounter in the registry exam, and we wouldn't want to do that if we could—the integrity of the exam is too important. *Vascular Technology Review* is not meant to be a Beat-the-SAT sort of book. It *is* meant to help you solidify your knowledge by giving you questions in the style of and with the content that you can expect on the registry. It gives you the opportunity to test yourself and to learn from the experience, building your confidence, identifying your strengths and weaknesses, and practicing your exam-taking skills so that you can better demonstrate your knowledge on the actual exam.

We welcome feedback, both positive and negative. If you find a questionable question— or answer—please let us know: info@daviespublishing.com is the e-mail address. We also want to know how you do on the exam. For your convenience, an evaluation form (*You Grade Us!*) appears in Part X.

I'd like to thank some folks for their help with this project:

- Pat, my wife, for putting up with me while I slogged through all this.

- Mike Davies, the publisher and editor, who was most patient with my slow progress and who had to tie up a bunch of the loose ends. Also Janet Heard of Davies Publishing, who had to clean the Augean stable of my manuscript.

- Barton Bean, Donna Cox, Keith Mauney, John Bennett, Colleen Douville, Andrew Hayes, Margaret Johnson, Ruth Kalmer-Holmes, Robert McGrath, Cynthia Ramirez, and Lars Shaw, whose fine work created the first three editions of the book that has helped literally thousands of RVTs pass their exams.

- Cindy Owen, who graciously contributed many of her own questions, answers, and always sterling explanations from her review book and courses. No good deed going unpunished, she has been credited as Special Contributor to this book.

- Polly deCann Wilson, who contributed some of the tips in *Coping with the Exam*, a collection of practical advice that follows this preface.

- MedaSonics and Advanced Technology Laboratories for their permission to use several useful images.

- And all the people at ARDMS, ICAVL, SVU, SDMS, and many other organizations who keep working to raise and maintain a level of excellence in this field.

Finally, you have not only our best wishes for success, but also our admiration for taking this big and important step in your career.

Don Ridgway

Donald P. Ridgway, RVT
El Cajon, California

Coping with the Exam

BEFORE THE EXAM

Study

Use flashcards

Join a study group

Take a review course

Wind down a week before

Don't cram

Relax

Study. And then study some more. Start early—six months in advance is reasonable, depending on how much free time you can devote to your preparation—and set a regular study schedule. Make your schedule specific so you know exactly what you must study on a particular day. Establish realistic goals so that you don't build a mountain you can't climb. Write it on your calendar, and stick to it.

As to *what* you study, don't just read aimlessly—use and refer to the sources in this book's bibliography and references. This book happens to be part two of a 3-step study program that covers and follows the very detailed ARDMS exam outline: (1) A concise, didactic, explanatory review of everything on the exam outline (*Vascular Technology: An Illustrated Review*, by Rumwell and McPharlin), (2) a mock exam based on the exam outline (this book), and (3) a flashcard drill that helps you memorize key facts and figures, think on your feet, and review the exam outline from a different angle (*ScoreCards for Vascular Technology*, by Owen and Strandness). This program offers a very reasonable, effective, and focused approach that concentrates your time and energy on the specific topics you must know to pass the exam and be a good technologist and sonographer. It also encourages you to familiarize yourself with and read other works, including the standard references, to read journal articles, and to poke around in the literature for specific bits of information that will deepen your knowledge of the facts and principles on which you will be tested.

Whether or not you use this particular program, or certain of its components, the approach is sound: Rely on a small core group of references, referring to others as necessary to firm up your understanding of specific topics. Use the exam outline to guide your studies. And use different but complementary study methods—texts, flashcards, and mock exams—to exercise those neural pathways.

Make and/or buy flashcards. Both is probably better, since the ones you buy may have questions you haven't thought of and because making your own reinforces your knowledge in a distinctly different way. Cindy Owen's and Dr. Strandness's *ScoreCards for Vascular Technology* is very effective and complement this book nicely. Doing your own 3 x 5 cards will help you organize and reinforce what you know as well. Again, study exercises using several complementary methods reinforce different neural pathways.

Study in a group. *This is very, very important.* You have blind spots, and the group can find and fix them. In addition, it is important to be able to articulate concepts, not just to pick out answers on a multiple-choice exam. Good vascular technologists and sonographers are also educators. Practice educating each other. Have sessions dedicated to specific content areas (such as "Venous Disease and Diagnosis"), and assign each group member some of the items from the exam outline. That way people are counting on you to bring something to the party, and you have to focus on your contribution. Weekly sessions are good.

Spend the bucks and take one of those review courses. This is a pretty good investment for most people at the stage of taking the ARDMS exam. First, think of it as insurance. Second, it's a nice way to consolidate your overall knowledge of the field, which many techs find valuable. In addition, you meet some other people in the field, and that's good by itself. Your clinical site might be willing to help with this expense. And you may be able to write it off; check with your accountant.

Ease down on the studying and stress the week before. If you've done a good job studying, you can safely wind down in your final week to reduce stress, build confidence, and rest up.

Breathe. In for a count of five through gently-pursed lips, then out for a count of five. Five times. There, isn't that better? Do this during the exam, too.

No studying the night before. You had your chance. Now just go to a really dumb movie and relax. Go to bed early and sleep well.

Organize your things the night before: Lay out comfortable clothes (including a sweater or sweatshirt in case the testing center is cold), pencils, your ARDMS test-admission papers, car and house keys, glasses, prescriptions, directions to the test center, and any other personal items you might need. You don't want to have to think that much the next day.

THE EXAM

Eat lightly, arrive early, avoid coffee

Take a sweater

Be confident!

Read each question twice

Answer the easy ones first

Guess—but wisely—when you have to

Pace yourself

Never despair

Take a deep breath

Eat lightly. You do not want to fall asleep during the exam.

Arrive early. Leave early enough to arrive at the test center early, especially if you haven't been there before. You don't need the added stress of a wrong-offramp adventure. Be sure to take directions, including the telephone number of the testing center in case you have to make contact en route.

Lay off the coffee. Guess how grim it gets if your bladder begins distracting you halfway through the exam. If you are a coffee or tea drinker, get up early enough to have a cup and visit the bathroom before leaving. Should you need to use the bathroom during the exam, don't worry. You can. You just have to notify the test proctor first.

Take a sweater. Sometimes it's bloody cold in those places, and you'll be a bit vasoconstricted anyway.

Be confident. Or at least affect a confident air. When you're waiting for the exam to begin, you should smile, lift both hands and wave them toward yourself, and say, "Bring it on." Welcome the challenge, because *you* are a smart tech, by golly.

Read each question twice before answering. Guess how easy it is to get one word wrong and misunderstand the whole question.

Try to answer the question without looking at the choices. Then look for your answer among the answer choices. This practice minimizes the distractibility of the incorrect answer choices, which in the test-making business are called—guess what?—*distractors*.

Knock off the easy ones first. Walk briskly through the exam and answer the questions you feel good about. Then go back through and answer the more difficult items. Next, one or two more passes to get the really tough ones. Finally, for those remaining

questions you just cannot answer with certainty, eliminate the obviously wrong answer choices and then guess (see below).

Don't second-guess. The common wisdom is that your first answer is more likely than revised answers to be correct, and that when you return to a question and change the answer, you'll probably be wrong. I don't know for sure that I agree. I know that I frequently rethink a question and realize I had something wrong to begin with. So, frankly, I include this obligatory bit of advice with a grain of salt. I guess you should change an answer only if you're quite sure you should.

Pace yourself; watch the time. I have known a few people to get so involved in the registry exam that they did not quite finish. Some tiresome folks fly through the exam in an hour and walk away whistling, but you should plan to take the whole time-allotment so you can work relaxed (or at least as un-tense as possible). If you feel good about finishing early, so be it.

Start winding it up 15 minutes before the end. Work methodically and quickly to make your best guesses at the gnarly ones, and leave no question unanswered or un-guessed-at.

If you have to guess, then guess. Passing the exam depends on the number of correct answers you make. Because unanswered questions are counted as *in*correct, it makes sense to guess when all else fails. The ARDMS itself advises that "it is to the candidate's advantage to answer all possible questions."

I hesitate to mention it, but there is a potentially handy book called *How to Beat the SAT* by Michael Donner. It takes you through different strategies for dealing with multiple-choice questions, from the ones you know cold to the ones that might as well be written in a Martian dialect. This is not to recommend cheating or faking it, but only to give people with severe test-anxiety a chance to cope. Among the hints in Donner's book:

- Eliminate the dumb answers, then the less-dumb answers, then work on the possibles, guessing, if necessary, at the correct answer. By eliminating obviously incorrect answers, you increase the odds that your final answer will be correct. If you were simply to guess at one out of five possible answers, you would have only a 20% chance of success. If, on the other hand, you use your knowledge and skill to eliminate three of the five answer choices, you increase your odds of success to 50%.

- Your best guess on a question in Martian (i.e., you have absolutely no idea what to make of it) is probably a B or a D, because A, C, and E are the most common guesses, so test-makers often avoid those. Nevertheless, second-guessing the test-makers can get rather tangled. Study instead.

Take notes on tricky or long questions. You can often help jog your memory or reasoning by rearranging the information in the question on your scratch paper.

Don't despair 50 minutes into the exam. At some point in the exam you may feel that things just aren't going well. Do the breathing for a minute (count of five in, count of five out) and plunge back in. You need only about three out of four correct answers to pass, and if you've put a reasonable amount of time into getting ready, that's attainable even if you feel sweat running down your back.

> Uncle Don says,
>
> **Don't forget to breathe!**

TAKING THE EXAM ON COMPUTER

Just point and click

Take notes

Mark and return to the hard questions

Use the on-screen clock to pace yourself

Be methodical

Breathe

Some candidates express concern about taking the registry exam on computer. Most folks find this to be pretty easy; some find it off-putting, at least in prospect. But the computerized exams are quite convenient: You can take the exam at your convenience (a far cry from the days of one exam per year), you know whether or not you passed before you leave the testing center (compare that to waiting weeks and even months, as used to be the case), and you can reschedule the exam after 90 days if you happen not to pass the first time (rather than waiting another six months to a year). Another good point: The illustrations are said to be clearer on computer than in the booklets on a Scantron-type exam.

Taking the test by computer is not complicated. The center even gives you a tutorial to be sure you know what you need to do. You sit in a carrel with a computer and answer the multiple-choice questions by pointing and clicking with a mouse. There is a clock on the display letting you know how much time is left. Use it to pace yourself. Scratch paper is available; make liberal use of it.

You can mark questions for answering later. A display shows which questions have not been answered so you can return to them. When you have finished, you click on "DONE," and you find out immediately whether you passed.

It's nothing to be afraid of. The principles are the same as those for any exam. Be methodical and keep breathing.

Thanks to Polly DeCann Wilson for some of the hints and advice about coping, taken from an old review-course syllabus.

Contents

PART I

Anatomy, Physiology & Hemodynamics

Cerebrovascular System
Venous System
Peripheral Arterial System
Abdominal / Visceral Vasculature
Microscopic Anatomy

CEREBROVASCULAR SYSTEM

Aortic arch

Upper extremity

Cervical carotid

Vertebral

Intracranial (circle of Willis)

1. The first major arterial branch of the aorta is the:

    A. Right common carotid artery
    B. The left common carotid artery
    C. The right subclavian artery
    D. The innominate artery
    E. The left subclavian artery

2. Which of the following arteries does NOT arise from the subclavian artery?

    A. Vertebral
    B. Superior thyroid
    C. Internal thoracic
    D. Thyrocervical trunk (axis)
    E. Internal mammary

3. The angular artery is the terminal part of the:

    A. Supraorbital artery
    B. Infraorbital artery
    C. Superficial temporal artery
    D. Transverse facial artery
    E. Facial artery

4.   The arterial pulsations felt in front of the ear and just above the zygomatic arch are from which artery?

   A. Maxillary
   B. Transverse facial
   C. Superficial temporal
   D. Facial
   E. Occipital

5.   The common carotid artery divides into its external and internal branches usually at the level of the upper border of the:

   A. Hyoid
   B. Cricoid
   C. Thyroid cartilage
   D. Cricothyroid membrane
   E. Carina

6.   What artery is usually the first branch of the external carotid artery?

   A. Inferior thyroid artery
   B. Superior thyroid artery
   C. Supraclavicular artery
   D. Facial artery
   E. Posterior auricular artery

7.   Which of the following is not an artery in the circle of Willis?

   A. Anterior cerebral artery
   B. Middle cerebral artery
   C. Anterior communicating artery
   D. Middle communicating artery
   E. Posterior communicating artery

8.   Which of the following arteries arise(s) from the external carotid artery?

   A. Superior thyroid artery
   B. Lingual artery
   C. Facial artery
   D. Ascending pharyngeal artery
   E. All the above

9.   The prominence of the larynx is formed by the:

   A. Hyoid bone
   B. Thyroid cartilage
   C. Cricoid cartilage
   D. Thyroid gland
   E. Greater cornu

10. The vertebral artery usually arises from the:

   A. Subclavian artery
   B. Thyrocervical trunk
   C. Costocervical trunk
   D. Superior thyroid artery
   E. Dorsal scapular artery

11. The infraorbital artery is a terminal branch of the:

   A. Maxillary artery
   B. Facial artery
   C. Inferior alveolar artery
   D. Transverse facial artery
   E. Superficial temporal artery

12. The vertebral arteries branch from the subclavian arteries to unite and form the:

   A. Ophthalmic artery
   B. Anterior cerebral artery
   C. Basilar artery
   D. Superficial temporal artery
   E. Posterior communicating artery

13. The first intracranial branch of the internal carotid artery is the:

   A. Superficial temporal artery
   B. Frontal artery
   C. Infraorbital artery
   D. Ophthalmic artery
   E. Middle cerebral artery

14. The circle of Willis receives its blood supply from which combination of arteries?

   A. Internal and external carotid arteries
   B. Subclavian and vertebral arteries
   C. Posterior cerebral artery and basilar artery
   D. Carotid and vertebral arteries
   E. Right and left vertebral arteries

15. The three terminal branches of the ophthalmic artery are the:

   A. Superficial, facial, and frontal arteries
   B. Nasal, frontal, and supraorbital arteries
   C. Basilar, anterior communicating, and posterior communicating arteries
   D. Vertebral, facial, and nasal arteries
   E. Nasal, frontal, and facial arteries

16. Two of the major branches of the external carotid arteries include the:

   A. Supraorbital and frontal arteries
   B. Internal maxillary and ophthalmic arteries

C. Superficial temporal and facial arteries

D. Vertebral and internal maxillary arteries

E. Supraorbital and middle cerebral arteries

17. Intracranial potential collateral arteries include all but the following:

    A. Anterior communicating artery
    B. Posterior communicating artery
    C. Superficial temporal artery
    D. Leptomeningeal pathways
    E. Rete mirable

18. Which of the following is NOT true regarding the internal carotid artery?

    A. Its first major branch is the ophthalmic artery.
    B. It supplies a high-resistance system.
    C. It supplies a low-resistance system.
    D. It is part of the anterior cerebral system.
    E. It originates at the carotid bifurcation.

19. The two arteries creating the bidirectional signal observed 60 to 65 mm deep during transcranial insonation of the temporal window are the:

    A. Posterior cerebral and anterior cerebral arteries
    B. Right and left vertebral arteries
    C. Middle cerebral and posterior cerebral arteries
    D. Middle cerebral and anterior cerebral arteries
    E. Right (or left) vertebral and right (or left) posterior inferior cerebral arteries

20. What is the most common anomaly of the circle of Willis?

    A. Absence of one of the middle cerebral arteries
    B. Duplication of the posterior communicating arteries
    C. Hypoplasia of the proximal segment of one of the anterior cerebral arteries
    D. Absence or hypoplasia of one or both of the communicating arteries
    E. Duplication of the middle cerebral arteries

21. Matching:

Proximal Vessel	Branch or Continuation of Vessel
A. Innominate	1. Internal Carotid
B. Subclavian	2. Subclavian
C. Common Carotid	3. Basilar
D. Vertebral	4. Superficial temporal
E. External Carotid	5. Vertebral

22. Helical flow with flow separation in the posterolateral aspect of the carotid bulb is a sign of:

    A. Normal flow dynamics
    B. Thrombosis
    C. Dissection

D. Stenosis

E. Intraplaque hemorrhage

23. The most common anatomic variant of the aortic arch is:

    A. A common origin of the innominate and left common carotid arteries
    B. Origin of the left vertebral artery from the aortic arch
    C. Origin of the right subclavian artery from the aortic arch
    D. Origin of the right common carotid artery from the aortic arch
    E. Duplication of the subclavian arteries

VENOUS SYSTEM

Upper extremity

Lower extremity

Central veins

24. The great saphenous vein:

    A. Originates along the medial dorsum of the foot
    B. Passes superiorly, anterior to the medial malleolus
    C. Is accompanied by the saphenous nerve
    D. Receives tributaries from all surfaces of the lower extremity
    E. All are correct

25. Which of the following is NOT correct regarding the great saphenous vein?

    A. It passes superiorly on the lateral side of the knee.
    B. It passes superiorly on the medial side of the thigh.
    C. It enters the common femoral vein.
    D. It extends distally to the dorsum of the foot.
    E. It has more valves in the calf than in the thigh.

26. The superficial vein that sends flow to the three main perforating veins of the distal calf is called:

    A. Small saphenous vein
    B. Posterior accessory vein
    C. Peroneal vein
    D. Perforator trunk vein
    E. Medial malleolar vein

27. The paratibial perforating veins (formerly Boyd's perforator) are located:

    A. In the lower calf
    B. In the distal thigh
    C. In the proximal thigh
    D. On the dorsum of the foot
    E. Below the knee

28. The left common iliac vein:

    A. Crosses anterior to the left common iliac artery just distal to the aortic bifurcation
    B. Crosses anterior to the right common iliac artery just distal to the aortic bifurcation
    C. Crosses posterior to the left common iliac artery just distal to the aortic bifurcation
    D. Crosses posterior to the right common iliac artery just distal to the aortic bifurcation
    E. Does not cross either common iliac artery

29. From this cross-sectional diagram of the thigh, reading from superficial to deep, identify the vessels marked:

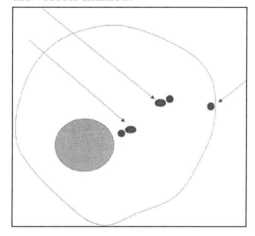

    A. Great saphenous vein, superficial femoral artery, profunda femoris artery
    B. Femoral vein, common femoral vein, common femoral artery
    C. Great saphenous vein, femoral vein, profunda femoris vein
    D. Superficial femoral artery, common femoral artery, deep femoral artery
    E. Great saphenous vein, superficial femoral artery, deep femoral vein

30. The brachial veins connect the:

    A. Ulnar and radial veins to the axillary vein
    B. Ulnar and radial veins to the subclavian vein
    C. Ulnar vein to the cephalic vein
    D. Radial vein to the subclavian vein
    E. Radial vein to the axillary vein

31. Of the following vein segments, which is imaged LEAST commonly?

    A. Distal femoral vein
    B. Proximal deep femoral vein
    C. Distal deep femoral vein
    D. Distal popliteal vein
    E. Common femoral vein

32. The term *muscle pump* refers to:

    A. The ventricles of the heart
    B. The right atrium of the heart
    C. The calf muscles
    D. The pulmonary arteries
    E. The veins in the groin

33. In this cross section of the calf, which letter represents the posterior tibial vessels?

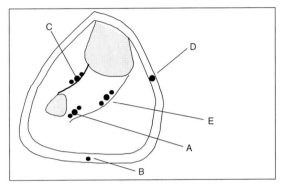

    A.
    B.
    C.
    D.
    E.

34. In this cross section, which letter represents the fibula?

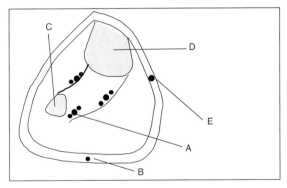

    A.
    B.
    C.
    D.
    E.

35. In this cross section, which letter represents the interosseous membrane?

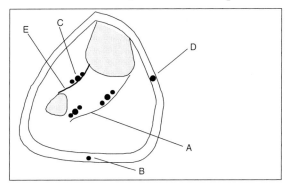

   A.
   B.
   C.
   D.
   E.

36. And in this same cross section, which letter represents the small saphenous vein?

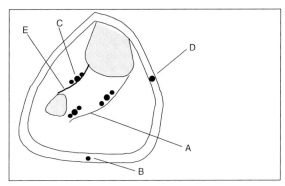

   A.
   B.
   C.
   D.
   E.

37. Which vein in the antecubital fossa connects the cephalic and basilic veins?

   A. Axillary vein
   B. Median cubital vein
   C. Cephalic vein
   D. Basilic vein
   E. Ulnar vein

38. Which of the following is NOT a deep vein of the upper extremity?

   A. Ulnar vein
   B. Cephalic vein
   C. Axillary vein
   D. Radial vein

E. Brachial vein

39. The brachiocephalic vein is found:

    A. Only on the right side
    B. Only on the left side
    C. On both the right and left sides
    D. There is no such vein; it is called "innominate"
    E. This vein is located centrally in the cranium

40. Which of the following vessels joins the brachial veins to form the axillary vein?

    A. Subclavian vein
    B. Innominate vein
    C. Cephalic vein
    D. Basilic vein
    E. Ulnar vein

41. Muscular veins of the calf that empty into the popliteal vein behind the knee are:

    A. Soleal sinuses
    B. Femoral veins
    C. Adductor veins
    D. Gastrocnemius veins
    E. Perforating veins

42. Compared to the arteries, veins have:

    A. Thicker, more muscular walls
    B. Thicker intima
    C. Thicker adventitia and media
    D. Thinner intima
    E. Thinner adventitia and media

43. Regarding venous valves, which is FALSE?

    A. Essential to muscle pump
    B. Bicuspid
    C. Endothelial tissue
    D. Allow flow only away from the heart
    E. Have sinuses to facilitate closure

PERIPHERAL ARTERIAL SYSTEM

Aortic arch

Upper extremity

Abdominal aorta

Lower extremity

44. Peripheral resistance increases with:

    A. Greater length, smaller diameter, and lower blood viscosity
    B. Greater length, larger diameter, and higher blood viscosity
    C. Shorter length, larger diameter, and lower blood viscosity
    D. Shorter length, smaller diameter, and lower blood viscosity
    E. Greater length, smaller diameter, and higher blood viscosity

45. The following arteries have low-resistance flow character:

    A. Internal carotid, preprandial superior mesenteric, and renal arteries
    B. External carotid, preprandial superior mesenteric, and renal arteries
    C. Internal carotid, postprandial superior mesenteric, and renal arteries
    D. External carotid, postprandial superior mesenteric, and renal arteries
    E. Internal carotid and superior mesenteric arteries

46. Which of the following statements about the dorsalis pedis artery is NOT correct?

    A. It runs anterior to the medial malleolus.
    B. It is typically the continuation of the anterior tibial artery.
    C. It joins the pedal arch about halfway along the dorsum of the foot.
    D. It is a branch of the peroneal artery.
    E. It begins at the bend of the foot and ankle.

47. Vessels and structures of the penis include all of the following EXCEPT:

    A. Deep artery of the penis
    B. Dorsal artery of the penis
    C. Corpus spongiosum
    D. Inferior vesicle artery
    E. Dorsal vein

48. Which of the following vessels is NOT found on or near the foot?

    A. The dorsalis pedis
    B. The posterior tibial
    C. The peroneal
    D. The circumflex
    E. All are found on or near the foot

49. In B-mode imaging of the common femoral artery and its bifurcation into the profunda femoris and superficial femoral arteries, normally the profunda femoris artery courses:

    A. Posterolateral to the superficial femoral artery
    B. Anterolateral to the superficial femoral artery
    C. Posteromedial to the superficial femoral artery
    D. Anteromedial to the superficial femoral artery
    E. Lateral to the superficial femoral artery

50. The popliteal trifurcation is actually a double bifurcation; select the pairs forming these two bifurcations:

    A. Posterior tibial and tibioperoneal trunk; then anterior tibial and peroneal
    B. Peroneal and tibioperoneal trunk; then posterior and anterior tibials
    C. Anterior tibial and popliteal; then posterior tibial and peroneal
    D. Posterior tibial and popliteal; then anterior tibial and peroneal
    E. Anterior tibial and tibioperoneal trunk; then posterior tibial and peroneal

51. The axillary artery connects the:

    A. Radial to the ulnar artery
    B. Ulnar to the brachial artery
    C. Brachial artery to the radial artery
    D. Radial to the subclavian artery
    E. Brachial artery to the subclavian artery

52. The great vessels arising from the aortic arch include all of the following EXCEPT the:

    A. Innominate artery
    B. Right subclavian artery
    C. Left common carotid artery
    D. Left subclavian artery
    E. All arise from the aortic arch

53. At the inguinal ligament, the external iliac artery becomes the:

    A. Internal iliac artery
    B. Profunda femoral artery
    C. Common femoral artery
    D. Superficial femoral artery
    E. Common iliac artery

54. This vessel courses along the medial aspect of the psoas muscle:

    A. Femoral artery
    B. Internal iliac artery
    C. External iliac artery
    D. Inferior mesenteric artery
    E. None of the above

ABDOMINAL & VISCERAL VASCULATURE

Arterial (celiac, mesenteric, renal, hepatic)

Venous (vena cava, renal, portal, mesenteric)

55. The renal arteries arise from the aorta:

    A. Laterally
    B. Inferiorly to the inferior mesenteric artery

    C. Posteriorly

    D. Superiorly to the superior mesenteric artery

    E. Anteriorly

56. Because of the location of the inferior vena cava, the left renal vein:

    A. Crosses anterior to the aorta inferior to the left renal artery

    B. Crosses posterior to the aorta proximal to the renal artery

    C. Crosses posterior to the aorta distal to the renal artery

    D. Does not cross the aorta

    E. Is displaced superior to the origin of the celiac axis

57. In a cross section of the aorta and surrounding regions, the vein that is visualized superficial to the aorta and the origins of the right and left renal arteries and deep to the superior mesenteric artery is the:

    A. Superior mesenteric vein

    B. Right renal vein

    C. Left renal vein

    D. Inferior mesenteric vein

    E. Celiac vein

58. The superior mesenteric artery typically originates from the:

    A. Aorta between the celiac trunk and the renal arteries

    B. Common mesenteric trunk or axis

    C. Aorta inferior to the renal arteries

    D. Aorta superior to the celiac trunk

    E. Celiac trunk

59. The superior vena cava is formed by the junction of the:

    A. Inferior vena cava and right innominate vein

    B. Innominate and right subclavian veins

    C. Innominate and left subclavian veins

    D. Right and left brachiocephalic veins

    E. Right and left subclavian veins

60. The portal vein is formed by the junction of the:

    A. Superior mesenteric and colic veins

    B. Inferior mesenteric and splenic veins

    C. Superior mesenteric and splenic veins

    D. Right and left hepatic veins

    E. Right and left portal veins

61. A useful landmark for locating the renal arteries is the:

    A. Superior mesenteric artery

    B. Right renal vein

    C. Celiac axis

    D. Common hepatic artery

E. Inferior mesenteric artery

62. The splenic, common hepatic, and left gastric arteries arise from this abdominal artery:

    A. Inferior mesenteric artery
    B. Proper hepatic artery
    C. Superior mesenteric artery
    D. Celiac trunk
    E. They are not branches of the same artery.

63. The most common anatomic variation of the renal arteries is:

    A. Congenital absence of one main renal artery
    B. Multiple renal arteries
    C. Anterocaval course of right renal artery
    D. Retroaortic renal artery
    E. Coarctation of the renal artery

64. Which artery supplies the small intestine, right colon, and transverse colon?

    A. Inferior mesenteric
    B. Superior mesenteric
    C. Left gastric
    D. Right gastric
    E. Gastroduodenal

65. Another name for the hypogastric artery is:

    A. External iliac artery
    B. Gastroduodenal artery
    C. Hepatic artery
    D. Internal iliac artery
    E. Celiac artery

66. Which artery is the left branch of the celiac trunk?

    A. Splenic artery
    B. Hepatic artery
    C. Left gastric artery
    D. Gastroduodenal artery
    E. The relative size of the branches varies too widely to say with certainty.

67. What is the name of the tiny intrarenal branches that arise from the interlobar arteries at right angles and course above the renal pyramids?

    A. Arcuate arteries
    B. Segmental arteries
    C. Interlobular arteries
    D. Capsular arteries
    E. Intralobular arteries

MICROSCOPIC ANATOMY

Arterial

Venous

68. The smallest vessels in the body are:

   A. Arterioles
   B. Venules
   C. Capillaries
   D. Intimas
   E. Adventitias

69. The term *tunica adventitia* denotes:

   A. The inner lining of the arterial wall
   B. The outer lining of the arterial wall
   C. Transverse arterial muscle fibers
   D. The intimal wall
   E. The middle layer of the arterial wall

70. The term *tunica intima* denotes:

   A. The inner lining of the arterial wall
   B. The outer lining of the arterial wall
   C. Transverse arterial muscle fibers
   D. Longitudinal muscle fibers
   E. The middle layer of the arterial wall

71. The blood supply to vascular tissue is provided by:

   A. Media perforators
   B. Vasa vasorum
   C. Osmosis across the intima only
   D. Septal capillary networks
   E. Tunica vasum

72. The layer of arterial or venous wall composed entirely of endothelial cells is the:

   A. Tunica adventitia
   B. Tunica media
   C. Tunica intima
   D. No layer is composed of only one type of tissue.
   E. Each layer is composed entirely of endothelial tissue.

73. Regarding capillaries, which is FALSE?

   A. They have only intima and adventitia layers.
   B. They measure approximately 8 microns in diameter
   C. The transit time of blood through capillaries is approximately one to three seconds.
   D. They lose fluid at the arteriolar end.
   E. They resorb fluid at the venular end.

74. A venule contains which vessel layers?

   A. Tunica adventitia, tunica media, and tunica intima
   B. Tunica adventitia and tunica media
   C. Tunica adventitia and tunica intima
   D. Tunica media and tunica intima
   E. Tunica media and tunica adventitia

PART II

Cerebrovascular Disease

Mechanisms of Cerebrovascular Disease
Signs and Symptoms of Cerebrovascular Disease
Testing and Treatment of Cerebrovascular Disease

MECHANISMS OF CEREBROVASCULAR DISEASE

Risk factors

Atherosclerosis

Dissection

Thromboembolism

Subclavian steal

Carotid body tumor

Fibromuscular dysplasia

Neointimal hyperplasia

75.　Atherosclerosis is a disease that begins in the:

A. Adventitia
B. Intima
C. Transverse fibers
D. Inner media
E. Outer media

76.　Which of the following is NOT considered a risk factor for atherosclerosis?

A. Hypertension
B. Female gender
C. Diabetes mellitus
D. Lipoprotein abnormalities
E. Tobacco use

77.　Which of the following is a complication of plaque ulceration?

A. Thrombosis
B. Intraplaque hemorrhage
C. Embolization
D. All of the above
E. None of the above

78. Cerebrovascular fibromuscular dysplasia occurs in:

    A. Males
    B. Females
    C. Australians
    D. Infants
    E. Hypoglycemics

79. Which of the following is NOT true regarding atherosclerosis?

    A. Atherosclerosis starts as a breakdown of the intima.
    B. Atherosclerosis usually develops at bifurcations.
    C. Atherosclerosis is a red blood cell disease.
    D. Atherosclerosis is a generalized disease.
    E. Intimal damage/repair may begin in adolescence.

80. A left arm blood pressure that is 40 mmHg lower than the right can be the result of any of the following EXCEPT:

    A. Thoracic outlet entrapment
    B. Subclavian steal
    C. Coarctation of the aortic arch
    D. Axillary artery embolus
    E. Innominate artery occlusion

81. With a subclavian artery stenosis on the right side:

    A. The flow in the right vertebral artery will be reversed.
    B. The patient will have right arm claudication.
    C. The arm pressure will be reduced.
    D. The right axillary artery Doppler signal will be monophasic.
    E. None of the above will necessarily be present.

82. Which of the following anatomic lesions can produce a vertebral steal?

    A. Innominate artery occlusion
    B. Left subclavian artery origin stenosis
    C. Left vertebral artery stenosis
    D. Right common carotid artery occlusion
    E. Right axillary artery occlusion
    F. D and E
    G. A and B

83. A hypertensive, diabetic 65-year old male presents for cerebrovascular testing because of an asymptomatic bruit on the right side. You are considering all of the following to be potential sources of the bruit EXCEPT:

    A. Stenosis of the external carotid artery
    B. Stenosis of the subclavian artery
    C. Occlusion of the common carotid artery
    D. Dissection of the common carotid artery
    E. All of the above may produce a bruit

84. A disease that affects primarily the intima and may extend into the media is:

    A. Buerger's disease
    B. Aneurysmal disease
    C. Atherosclerosis
    D. Takayasu's disease
    E. Diabetes

85. After carotid bifurcation disease, the next most common source of stroke symptoms is:

    A. Cardiac-source embolization
    B. Paradoxical embolization from DVT via patent foramen ovale
    C. Spinal stenosis
    D. Subclavian stenosis
    E. Aortic dissection

86. The strongest risk factor for stroke is:

    A. Poor diet
    B. Obesity
    C. Hypertension
    D. Hypocholesterolemia
    E. Alcohol abuse

87. In the cerebrovascular system, atherosclerosis occurs most commonly in the:

    A. Origin of internal carotid artery
    B. Intracranial internal carotid artery
    C. Left subclavian artery
    D. Innominate artery
    E. Proximal common carotid artery

88. The most prevalent type of stroke is:

    A. Aneurysmal
    B. Hemorrhagic
    C. Septic embolic
    D. Venous thrombotic
    E. Ischemic

89. Where are carotid body tumors located?

    A. Medial to the origin of the external carotid artery
    B. Within the internal jugular vein
    C. Between the internal and external carotid arteries
    D. In the submandibular gland
    E. In the intracranial internal carotid artery

90. Which statement about subclavian steal is FALSE?

    A. It occurs most commonly on the left side.
    B. Most patients are asymptomatic.
    C. It results from severe stenosis or occlusion of the proximal vertebral artery.
    D. Lower blood pressure is seen in the affected arm.
    E. All of these statements are false.

91. A 24-year-old patient with a history of recent automobile accident arrives in the ICU with symptoms of acute right-side weakness and aphasia. The most likely etiology of these symptoms is:

    A. Carotid dissection
    B. Cerebral aneurysm rupture
    C. Severe internal carotid artery stenosis
    D. Embolic activity from cardiac mural thrombus
    E. Thrombocytopenia

92. A patient undergoes carotid endarterectomy. Six months later angiography is performed because of symptoms referable to the other side. The angiogram reveals that the operated carotid is significantly narrowed. The most likely cause is:

    A. Atherosclerotic plaque recurrence
    B. Carotid dissection
    C. Embolic activity
    D. Extrinsic compression
    E. Neointimal hyperplasia

SIGNS & SYMPTOMS OF CEREBROVASCULAR DISEASE

Transient symptoms

Stroke

Physical examination (neurology, bruits, bilateral brachial pressures)

93. The term *hemiparesis* means:

    A. Paralysis of one side
    B. Weakness of one side
    C. Numbness/tingling on one side
    D. Spasm of voluntary muscle on one side
    E. Dizziness

94. The NASCET (North American Symptomatic Carotid Endarterectomy Trial) used the following arteriographic criterion/criteria to classify internal carotid artery disease:

    A. Area and diameter stenoses calculated by dividing the minimal area and diameter at the internal carotid artery by the area and diameter at the common carotid artery.
    B. Area percentage stenosis calculated by dividing the minimal area by the original area at the site of stenosis.

C. Diameter percentage stenosis calculated by dividing the minimal diameter by the original diameter at the site of stenosis.

D. Diameter percentage stenosis calculated by dividing the minimal diameter by the diameter of the un-stenosed distal internal carotid artery.

E. Area percentage stenosis calculated by dividing the minimal area by the normal area of the distal internal carotid artery.

95. All of the following may represent symptoms from the brain stem or posterior circulation EXCEPT:

    A. Dizziness
    B. Vertigo
    C. Ectasia
    D. Syncope
    E. Amaurosis fugax

96. *[If true, check "True." If false, insert correct term.]* A patient relates a 10-minute episode of loss of vision. He closed each eye and the reduction in the right half of his visual field was present bilaterally. This patient is describing amaurosis fugax.

    True ( ) False _____

97. A symptom of vertebrobasilar insufficiency is:

    A. Unilateral paresis
    B. Aphasia
    C. Amaurosis fugax
    D. Diplopia
    E. None of the above

98. *[If true, check "True." If false, insert correct term.]* On ophthalmologic examination, a bright yellow spot is noted within a branch artery. This is a Hollenhorst plaque.

    True ( ) False _____

99. A patient complains of a temporary shading of the vision in one eye. This symptom is called:

    A. Subclavian steal syndrome
    B. Dysphasia
    C. Reversible ischemic neurologic event
    D. Amaurosis fugax
    E. Permanent ischemic neurologic event

100. The incidence of new strokes per year is:

    A. 150,000
    B. 250,000
    C. 500,000
    D. 1,000,000
    E. 2,600,000

101. The abbreviation *TIA* stands for:

    A. Terminal internal artery
    B. Temporary ischemic attack
    C. Transient ischemic attack
    D. Transient internal artery
    E. Temporary internal attack

102. A TIA of the right anterior hemisphere of the brain will likely affect:

    A. The entire body
    B. The left side of the body
    C. The right side of the body
    D. The right side of the face
    E. The back of the head

103. Amaurosis fugax related to an internal carotid lesion will cause:

    A. Permanent blindness of the contralateral eye
    B. Temporary blindness or shading of the ipsilateral eye
    C. Permanent blindness of the ipsilateral eye
    D. Temporary blindness or shading of the contralateral eye
    E. Temporary blindness or shading of both eyes

104. A transient ischemic attack:

    A. Resolves within 24 hours
    B. Does not resolve within 24 hours
    C. Resolves within 72 hours
    D. Resolves after 24 hours
    E. Resolves in one week

105. Simultaneous bilateral ocular symptoms in the patient with suspected cerebrovascular disease generally originate from:

    A. The vertebrobasilar arteries
    B. The ophthalmic arteries
    C. Both common carotid arteries
    D. Both internal carotid arteries
    E. Both external carotid arteries

106. Which of the following is a vertebrobasilar symptom?

    A. Aphasia
    B. Vertigo
    C. Amaurosis fugax
    D. Right anterior hemisphere TIA
    E. Unilateral paresis

107. Which one of the following is an anterior circulation symptom?

    A. Ataxia

    B. Drop attack

    C. Syncope

    D. Binocular visual disturbance

    E. Facial asymmetry

108. Which of the following accurately defines *RIND*, also called *stroke with recovery*?

    A. A reversible ischemic neurologic deficit that completely resolves within 24 hours.

    B. A neurologic deficit that does not resolve.

    C. A neurologic deficit that waxes and wanes.

    D. An irreversible neurologic deficit.

    E. A neurologic ischemic deficit that resolves completely after 24 hours.

109. A 56-year-old patient reports loss of vision in her left eye two days ago, with total resolution in 10 minutes. Yesterday morning she developed weakness and numbness in her right hand and was unable to hold her coffee cup. This afternoon her hand strength is about 90% normal, with normal sensation. Clinically she has:

    A. Amaurosis fugax

    B. Transient ischemic attack

    C. Migraine

    D. Stroke

    E. Lacunar infarct

110. Amaurosis fugax can be interpreted as a:

    A. Stroke of the visual cortex

    B. Transient ischemic attack

    C. Stroke of the eye

    D. Transient ischemic attack of the frontal cortex

    E. Stroke of the parietal cortex

111. Dysphagia is a:

    A. Hormone imbalance causing loss of appetite

    B. Psychological, not physiological, problem

    C. Left-hemisphere symptom (if patient is right-handed)

    D. Right-hemisphere symptom (if patient is right-handed)

    E. Symptom associated with vertebrobasilar insufficiency

112. A binocular disturbance that disrupts vision in half the visual field of both eyes is called:

    A. Hemiplegia

    B. Amaurosis duplex

    C. Dysphagia

    D. Homonymous hemianopia

    E. Hemiparesis

113. *Paresthesia* refers to:

    A. Dizziness

    B. Disturbance of speech

    C. Loss of function of a limb

    D. Weakness

    E. Tingling sensation

114. A patient describes a 30-minute episode of garbled speech. This is called:

    A. Dysphasia

    B. Aphasia

    C. Paresthesia

    D. Dysphagia

    E. Syncope

115. The patient in the previous question is right-handed. Which area of circulation is suspect?

    A. Right hemisphere

    B. Left hemisphere

    C. Occipital cortex

    D. Vertebrobasilar territory

    E. Brainstem circulation

116. Which of the following is true regarding subclavian steal?

    A. Resulting strokes are usually severely disabling.

    B. It is usually a harmless hemodynamic phenomenon.

    C. It is caused by arterial obstruction proximal to the origin of the vertebral artery.

    D. It is caused by arterial obstruction distal to the origin of the vertebral artery.

    E. A and C

    F. A and D

    G. B and C

    H. B and D

117. Subclavian steal occurs:

    A. More often on the right side

    B. More often on the left side

    C. Equally often on both sides

    D. Mainly in young, male smokers

    E. Mainly in females

118. A hemispheric stroke usually affects:

    A. The anterior cerebral artery distribution and the ipsilateral side of the body

    B. The middle cerebellar artery distribution and the ipsilateral side of the body

    C. The external carotid distribution, and may affect one or both sides of the body

    D. The anterior cerebellar artery distribution and the contralateral side of the body

    E. The middle cerebral artery distribution and the contralateral side of the body

119. Stenosis of the following vessel presents the highest risk for a TIA:

    A. Left main coronary artery

    B. Common carotid artery

    C. Internal carotid artery

D. External carotid artery

E. Middle cerebral artery

120. A decreased pulse at mid neck is suggestive of:

   A. Carotid aneurysm

   B. Common carotid stenosis if the contralateral pulse is normal

   C. Common carotid stenosis if the contralateral pulse is decreased

   D. Internal carotid stenosis if the contralateral pulse is normal

   E. Internal carotid stenosis if the contralateral pulse is also decreased

121. Which is NOT true regarding carotid bruit?

   A. Severe stenosis may cause a bruit.

   B. The absence of a bruit rules out significant stenosis.

   C. The presence of a bruit is significant.

   D. A cervical bruit might arise from stenosis of the external carotid artery.

   E. A bruit extending into diastole suggests severe stenosis.

122. Bruits heard bilaterally, loudest low in the neck, are most likely caused by:

   A. Aortic valve stenosis

   B. Innominate stenosis

   C. Bilateral subclavian stenosis

   D. Aortic arch occlusion

   E. Bilateral CCA obstruction

123. A stronger pulse is palpated in the right neck than on the left. This could result from all of the following EXCEPT:

   A. Tortuous CCA

   B. Carotid aneurysm on the right

   C. Tech error

   D. Left carotid obstruction

   E. Innominate occlusion

124. Which of the following is/are TRUE regarding the clinical detection of a bruit?

   A. A bruit is always an indication of disease.

   B. It means that turbulent flow exists.

   C. It may be indicative of valvular dysfunction in the heart.

   D. It may be a normal finding in parts of some vessels and during periods of enhanced flow.

   E. A bruit is present in >90% of vessels with disease.

   F. B, C, and D.

   G. A, B, and E.

125. During ordinary auscultation of a carotid bifurcation, the detection of a bruit that extends into diastole is:

   A. Insignificant

   B. Marginally significant

    C. Moderately significant

    D. Highly significant

    E. Impossible

126. Which of these conditions is LEAST likely to cause a bruit in the neck?

    A. Severe stenosis of the internal carotid artery

    B. Severe stenosis of the external carotid artery

    C. Hyperdynamic carotid flows

    D. Cardiac valvular disease

    E. Critical preocclusive stenosis of the internal carotid artery

127. Why are brachial blood pressures obtained bilaterally when evaluating a patient for cerebrovascular disease?

    A. The systolic components from each arm are averaged to determine the likelihood of cerebrovascular disease.

    B. It is necessary to know both brachial pressures to rule out the presence of hypoperfusion syndrome.

    C. The brachial blood pressures are compared to see if they are equal.

    D. Both brachial blood pressures must be known to determine if hypertension is present.

    E. There is no value in obtaining bilateral brachial pressures if they are not compared to the ankle pressures.

TESTING & TREATMENT OF CEREBROVASCULAR DISEASE

    Noninvasive testing (patient positioning, technique, interpretation, capabilities, limitations)

    Duplex imaging (B-mode, Doppler, color Doppler)

    Transcranial Doppler

    Miscellaneous diagnostic tests (methods, interpretation, limitations)

    Arteriography

    MR angiography

    CT

    Treatment and follow-up (medical, endovascular, surgical)

128. All of the following statements apply to pulsed-wave Doppler EXCEPT:

    A. Aliasing occurs when the frequency shift exceeds ½ the pulse repetition frequency.

    B. One transducer is used for both transmission and reception.

    C. The beam is continuously transmitted with intermittent reception according to vessel depth.

    D. A sample volume is used to determine the depth of interest.

    E. All of these statements are true.

129. Loss of the spectral window with pulsed Doppler ultrasound occurs with:

    A. Flow turbulence

    B. Parabolic flow
    C. Laminar flow
    D. All of the above
    E. None of the above

130. A duplex image of the carotid bifurcation that demonstrates a goblet-like configuration of the internal and external branches curving around a highly vascularized mass suggests:

    A. Carotid aneurysm
    B. Severe ICA stenosis
    C. Myointimal hyperplasia
    D. Carotid body tumor
    E. Temporal arteritis

131. In duplex imaging, the best arterial wall image quality is obtained when the beam is at the following angle to the artery walls:

    A. 90°
    B. 60°
    C. 0°
    D. Oblique
    E. Obtuse

132. TCD findings consistent with vasospasm following subarachnoid hemorrhage would include:

    A. Absence of diastolic flow in the middle cerebral artery
    B. Greatly diminished diastolic flow in the middle cerebral artery
    C. Retrograde flow in the middle cerebral artery
    D. Greatly increased mean velocities in the middle cerebral artery
    E. This is not a condition for which TCD is a useful modality.

133. In TCD, the normal direction of flow in the vertebral artery is:

    A. Toward the beam
    B. Away from the beam
    C. Bidirectional
    D. Dependent on the cardiac cycle
    E. Not detectable with TCD

134. Which of the following is NOT a condition for which TCD might be useful?

    A. Vasospasm following subarachnoid hemorrhage
    B. Determination of brain death
    C. Cerebral artery monitoring during surgery
    D. Carotid siphon stenosis
    E. Temporal arteritis

135. The Doppler beam angle considered optimal for standardization of duplex carotid studies at most vascular labs is:

    A. 0°

    B. 20–40°

    C. 40–45°

    D. 60°

    E. Any angle greater than 60°

136. The usual instrumentation for handheld TCD includes a probe with an operating frequency of:

    A. 10 KHz

    B. 2 MHz

    C. 5 MHz

    D. 7.5 MHz

    E. 10 MHz

137. In TCD, the normal direction of flow in the anterior cerebral artery is:

    A. Toward the beam

    B. Away from the beam

    C. Bidirectional

    D. Dependent on the cardiac cycle

    E. Not detectable with TCD

138. A localized increase in mean velocity from 50 to 150 cm/sec at a depth of 50 mm with the TCD transducer placed in the temporal window probably indicates:

    A. Significant stenosis of the anterior cerebral artery

    B. Moderate generalized vasospasm

    C. Significant stenosis of the internal carotid at the siphon

    D. Significant vasospasm of the middle cerebral artery

    E. Significant stenosis of the middle cerebral artery

139. In handheld TCD, the angle of the beam relative to flow is assumed to be:

    A. 0°

    B. 30°

    C. 45° exactly

    D. 60°

    E. 90°

140. You perform TCD, insonating the left anterior cerebral artery. The flow is toward the beam. This finding suggests:

    A. Ipsilateral carotid obstruction, with right-to-left collateralization.

    B. Contralateral carotid obstruction, with left-to-right collateralization.

    C. Ipsilateral carotid obstruction, with posterior-to-anterior collateralization.

    D. Contralateral siphon disease.

    E. Nothing of diagnostic significance.

141. Which of the following would alter the frequency shift of the internal carotid artery Doppler signal?

    A. Tapering of the vessel from the bulb to the distal visualized segment

B. Increasing the transmitted frequency
C. Readjusting the angle-correct cursor
D. Lowering the system threshold sensitivity
E. A and B
F. C and D

142. Which one of the following diagnostic criteria for stenosis would be anticipated in the presence of a 50–60% diameter stenosis of the internal carotid artery?

A. Poststenotic turbulence only
B. Blunting of the systolic waveform with absence of a diagnostic frequency, at the site of maximum frequency shift change
C. Elevation of both systolic and diastolic frequency components, with minimal poststenotic turbulence
D. Elevation of systolic and diastolic frequency components with no demonstrable poststenotic turbulence
E. Elevation of systolic frequency with poststenotic turbulence

143. The best way to prepare a transducer for intraoperative use is:

A. Autoclave it.
B. Immerse it in Cidex solution for 72 hours.
C. Wash it with soap and water.
D. Place transducer and acoustic gel within a sterile sleeve or bag.
E. Microwave it.

144. In using continuous-wave Doppler with spectral analysis to assess the internal carotid artery, which of the following operator-induced errors would most likely result in a falsely LOW frequency shift?

A. Overdriving the Doppler signal gain
B. Allowing the signal beam to overlap both an artery and a vein
C. Changing to a higher-frequency transducer
D. Leaving the wall filter on
E. Increasing the beam angle to 70°

145. Of the chief advantages of continuous-wave Doppler, which of the following is FALSE?

A. Aliasing cannot occur; recording of extremely high frequency shifts is possible.
B. It allows more precise range-gating than pulsed-wave Doppler.
C. The signal-to-noise ratio is inherently greater than pulsed Doppler systems due to its continuous state of operation.
D. Continuous-wave Dopplers are less expensive.
E. The instrumentation is less complex than in pulsed-wave Doppler.

146. Among the chief limitations of continuous-wave Doppler is (are):

A. Depth information is not possible; precise location of flow pattern cannot be determined.
B. The two-transducer system is inherently more expensive.

C. Polarity of the reflected signal frequency shift cannot be determined; direction of blood flow cannot be defined.

D. FFT spectral analysis cannot be applied to continuous-wave Doppler signal information.

E. The sample volume is too small to interrogate deeper vessels.

147. Which of the following statements about this figure is TRUE?

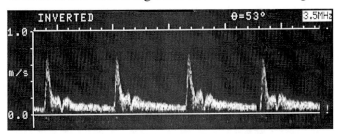

A. This spectrum is characteristic of an external carotid artery.
B. This spectrum is characteristic of a common carotid artery.
C. This spectrum is characteristic of an internal carotid artery.
D. This spectrum is severely stenotic in character.
E. This spectrum suggests distal total occlusion.

148. Which of the following is true regarding the spectrum below?

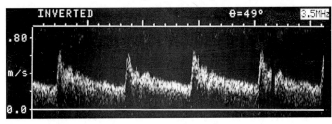

A. This spectrum is characteristic of an external carotid artery.
B. This spectrum is characteristic of a common carotid artery.
C. This spectrum is characteristic of an internal carotid artery.
D. This spectrum shows total window filling.
E. This spectrum suggests high distal resistance.

149. Which of the following statements is FALSE regarding the ICA spectrum below?

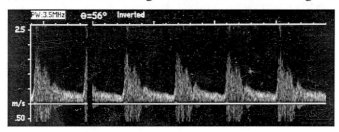

    A. There is forward flow throughout diastole.
    B. This appears to be from a low-resistance system.
    C. The absence of a systolic window in this spectrum indicates turbulent blood flow.
    D. The velocities indicate a hemodynamically significant stenosis.
    E. The velocities suggest severe (greater than 80%) stenosis.

150. The ICA waveform below has a peak-systolic velocity of 285 cm/sec, with an end-diastolic velocity of 66 cm/sec. Which of the following is/are true regarding this waveform?

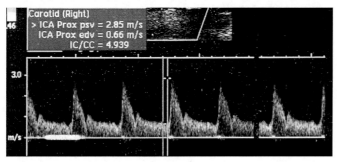

    A. This is within normal limits.
    B. The open systolic window suggests mild-to-moderate stenosis (<50% by diameter).
    C. The elevated peak-systolic velocities and significant end-diastolic velocities suggest significant ICA stenosis (>50% diameter).
    D. The severely elevated peak-systolic velocities and end-diastolic velocities suggest severe ICA stenosis (>80%).
    E. B and D.

151. In TCD, the normal direction of flow in the middle cerebral artery is:

    A. Toward the beam
    B. Away from the beam
    C. Bidirectional
    D. Dependent on the cardiac cycle
    E. Not detectable with TCD

152. Which of the following determinants dictate(s) transducer frequency selection for optimal carotid B-mode imaging?

    A. Desired beam width
    B. The average and extreme depths of carotid vessels in most subjects to be studied
    C. Desired axial resolution
    D. Cost
    E. A, B, and C

F. C and D

153. Which of the following imaging transducer frequencies could appropriately be used for assessment of the carotid arteries?

A. 10 MHz
B. 5 MHz
C. 2.5 MHz
D. 0.3 MHz
E. A and B

154. Which of the following is (are) true regarding axial resolution in carotid imaging?

A. Differentiates soft plaque from blood
B. Resolves two targets positioned one in front of another along the axis of beam propagation
C. Improves the observer's ability to estimate vessel wall thickness
D. Determines the absolute depth of penetration of ultrasound beam at a given frequency
E. A and D
F. B and C
G. B and D

155. Using the temporal window for TCD, you find a strong signal with considerable diastolic flow at a depth of 50 mm. This is most likely:

A. Anterior cerebral artery
B. Posterior cerebral artery
C. Middle cerebral artery
D. Vertebral artery
E. Basilar artery

156. To optimize carotid vessel image data, lateral resolution should be:

A. As small as possible, to differentiate calcified lesions from fresh thrombus
B. As small as possible, to resolve side-by-side lesions
C. As small as possible, to determine vessel wall and plaque thickness
D. As large as possible, to identify hemodynamically significant lesions
E. As large as possible for optimal sample volume placement

157. The TCD window used for assessing the middle cerebral artery is:

A. Temporal
B. Suboccipital
C. Orbital
D. Submandibular
E. Nasal

158. A carotid bruit can be detected with color flow and spectral analysis as:

A. A mosaic of low red and blue frequencies in color flow in tissue lying outside of the lumen, and oscillatory waveforms above and below baseline in the spectral waveform.

B. A mosaic of high red and blue aliasing frequencies in color flow and oscillatory waveforms above and below baseline in the spectral waveform.

C. A mosaic of high red and blue aliasing frequencies in color flow; bruits cannot appear on the spectral waveform.

D. A mosaic of low red and blue frequencies in color flow; bruits cannot appear on the spectral waveform.

E. High-frequency oscillations in the spectral waveform; bruits cannot appear on color flow.

159. All of the following are consistent with total occlusion of the internal carotid artery EXCEPT the:

A. Absence of flow in the ICA lumen
B. Decreased velocity proximal to occlusion
C. Retrograde flow in the distal internal carotid artery
D. Increase in flow through collateral pathways
E. Inability to be reconstructed surgically

160. This ultrasound image shows an internal carotid artery with:

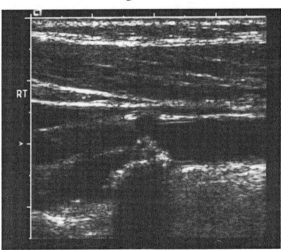

A. A calcified plaque
B. An ulcerated lesion
C. A normal arterial wall
D. An intraplaque hemorrhage
E. A homogeneous plaque

161. The following ultrasound image shows an internal carotid artery with:

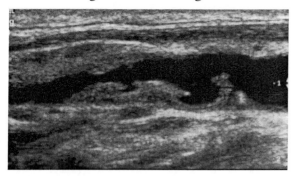

    A. Abnormal internal carotid artery wall
    B. A calcified plaque on the posterior wall
    C. A heterogeneous plaque
    D. A homogenous plaque
    E. An intraplaque hemorrhage

162. The TCD window used for assessing the ophthalmic artery and carotid siphon is:

    A. Temporal
    B. Suboccipital
    C. Orbital
    D. Submandibular
    E. Nasal

163. The Doppler diagnostic criterion that is most important for calling greater than 80% stenosis is:

    A. Mean or time-average velocity
    B. Peak-systolic velocity
    C. End-diastolic velocity
    D. Minimum mid-diastolic average velocity
    E. Percent window reduction

164. An arterial stenosis that is 75% by cross-sectional area reduction corresponds to a diameter reduction of:

    A. 75%
    B. 96%
    C. 60%
    D. 50%
    E. 35%

165. An arterial stenosis that is 80% by diameter reduction corresponds to a cross-sectional area reduction of:

    A. 96%
    B. 88%
    C. 70%
    D. 60%
    E. 45%

166. A vascular lab calls a stenosis 60–70% by diameter based on its duplex assessment, but angiography the next day calls it 90% by diameter. Possible reasons for this discrepancy might include all EXCEPT:

    A. The stenosis is long and smooth, changing its Doppler character compared to that of a shorter lesion.
    B. Only one plane of visualization was used for angiography.
    C. Poor angle-correction with the duplex, creating artificially low velocity estimates.
    D. Acoustic shadowing prevented Doppler assessment of the maximal narrowing.
    E. Color flow PRF set too low, creating aliasing and overestimation of velocities.

167. You are examining hardcopy of a TCD exam. One printout shows a spectral waveform labeled "suboccipital window," and the depth is indicated to be 90 mm. This is most likely the:

    A. Anterior cerebral artery
    B. Posterior cerebral artery
    C. Middle cerebral artery
    D. Vertebral artery
    E. Basilar artery

168. The characteristics of flow in the different carotid artery segments are:

    A. Low-resistance character in the ECA, high-resistance in the ICA, with mixed character in the CCA
    B. High-resistance character in the ECA, low-resistance in the ICA, with mixed character in the CCA
    C. Low-resistance in both the ICA and ECA, with higher-resistance character in the CCA
    D. High-resistance in both the ICA and ECA, with lower-resistance character in the CCA
    E. Low-resistance character throughout

169. The Doppler sample volume is usually adjusted:

    A. Small, to sample flow only from center stream
    B. Small, to sample flow right against the arterial walls
    C. Big enough to sample flow from the entire lumen of the artery
    D. Big enough to sample flow from a long segment of the artery
    E. Is not an issue with pulsed-wave Doppler

170. The angle-correct cursor for velocity estimates is best:

    A. Adjusted parallel with arterial walls
    B. Adjusted perpendicular to arterial walls
    C. Adjusted 0° throughout for maximum frequency shift
    D. Adjusted 60° at all times regardless of vessel direction
    E. Left off to avoid measurement errors

171. The components of information on the spectral Doppler display include all EXCEPT:

    A. Pixel brightness, indicating how many red blood cells are reflecting at a given frequency shift

    B. Frequency shift on the y-axis

    C. Time on the x-axis

    D. Depth on the y-axis

    E. All of the above are components of the spectral Doppler display.

172. Choose the color box that will NOT produce a reasonably good color display for this diving internal carotid artery.

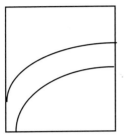

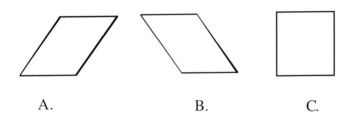

    A.   B.   C.

    D. None will produce good color.

    E. All will produce good color.

173. You are using color flow to scan an internal carotid artery that dives steeply distally, as shown. The color gets much brighter, even aliasing, in the distal portion of the artery. This probably means:

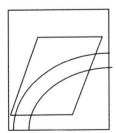

    A. The velocities are accelerating as the blood flows downhill.

    B. The frequency shifts are changing at different points in the color box due to the curvature of the artery.

    C. There is a significant stenosis distally causing the brighter color and aliasing.

    D. The color box should be angled in the opposite direction.

    E. It is not really the internal carotid but the external carotid artery.

174. You perform percussion maneuvers on the superficial temporal artery and see oscillations on the spectral display. The artery being insonated is most likely:

    A. Internal carotid artery
    B. External carotid artery
    C. Vertebral artery
    D. Thyrocervical trunk
    E. A low-resistance artery

175. Which of the following is NOT a useful color flow adjustment in an effort to detect slow flow in a possibly occluded internal carotid artery?

    A. Increase color flow gain
    B. Increase color flow PRF
    C. Decrease color flow PRF
    D. Decrease color flow wall filter
    E. Decrease beam angle relative to the vessel

176. Which of the following is NOT a duplex indication of a totally occluded internal carotid artery?

    A. ICA lumen filled with heterogeneous echoes
    B. No Doppler or color flow obtainable within ICA lumen
    C. Absence of diastolic flow in CCA spectral display
    D. Greatly increased end-diastolic velocities in CCA spectral display
    E. "Drumbeat" or "slapping" Doppler signal at ICA origin

177. This waveform from the left vertebral artery is:

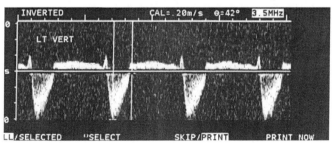

    A. Within normal limits
    B. Suggestive of ICA obstruction
    C. Suggestive of developing subclavian steal
    D. Suggestive of left brachial artery obstruction
    E. Monophasic

178. During a cerebrovascular exam, you obtain equal brachial systolic pressures bilaterally. During the scan, you obtain this pulsatile signal from between the transverse processes. You move the beam to the common carotid artery, and the waveform is below the baseline:

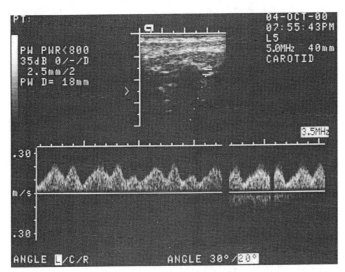

A. This waveform suggests antegrade vertebral artery flow.
B. This waveform is suggestive of left-side subclavian steal.
C. This waveform is suggestive of left internal carotid obstruction.
D. You should ask the patient to perform a Valsalva maneuver.
E. You should change to a lower-frequency transducer.

179. The acoustic windows through which ultrasound may pass in performing transcranial Doppler and transcranial imaging examinations include all except:

A. The temporal bone
B. The medial part of the frontal bone
C. The orbit of the eye
D. The suboccipital window
E. The submandibular area

180. Of the following, which is NOT one of the main collateral pathways in the event of ICA obstruction?

A. Posterior to anterior
B. Genicular to arcuate branches
C. Contralateral hemisphere
D. ECA branches to ophthalmic branches
E. All represent major cerebrovascular collateral pathways.

181. When visualizing the carotid bifurcation using duplex ultrasound, magnetic resonance imaging, or angiography, the best way to determine whether you are looking at the internal carotid is by the fact that:

A. The internal carotid has a bulb and the external carotid does not.
B. The external carotid has branches near the bifurcation and the internal carotid does not.
C. The internal carotid has branches near the bifurcation and the external carotid does not.
D. The external carotid has a smaller lumen than the internal carotid.
E. The internal carotid tapers at the bifurcation.

182. Conventional arteriography reveals 30% diameter stenosis in a symptomatic patient with severe stenosis by B-mode and peak systolic velocities of 250 cm/sec in the proximal internal carotid artery. Which of the following statements about these findings is TRUE?

    A. The high velocities were caused by carotid kinking.
    B. Even double-projection arteriography may fail to fully determine diameter stenosis, especially in the event of vessel overlap.
    C. Arteriography may fail to reveal small "berry" aneurysms in the brain.
    D. B-mode "plaquing" may have been background ultrasound noise.
    E. The ultrasound findings are not as important as the findings of an arch study.

183. Major complications of cerebrovascular angiography include all of the following EXCEPT:

    A. Death
    B. Stroke
    C. Inadvertent venous puncture
    D. Arterial occlusion at the access site
    E. Renal failure

184. Major complications of cerebrovascular angiography occur in approximately:

    A. 10% of patients
    B. 1% of patients
    C. 0.1% of patients
    D. 0.01% of patients
    E. >20% of patients

185. What information CANNOT be determined by cerebrovascular angiography?

    A. Degree of narrowing of ICA by diameter
    B. Presence of ulceration
    C. Degree of narrowing of ICA by cross-sectional area
    D. Total occlusion of ICA
    E. Crossover collateralization from the contralateral hemisphere

186. Angiography is generally considered only when the information is necessary for surgery or other urgent patient management because of all of these factors EXCEPT:

    A. It is expensive.
    B. It carries a risk of stroke.
    C. It carries a risk of anaphylactic complications.
    D. It is often nondiagnostic.
    E. It is an invasive procedure.

187. The most common arterial puncture site for all forms of angiography (including cerebral) is the:

    A. Common femoral artery
    B. Brachial artery
    C. Axillary artery
    D. Dorsal artery
    E. It depends on the area of the body being studied.

188. Advantages of angiography over duplex carotid studies include all EXCEPT:

    A. Ability to visualize intracranial collaterals
    B. Superiority at calling ulceration
    C. Ability to visualize the entire cerebral vasculature
    D. Unlimited repeatability
    E. Ability to determine siphon stenosis

189. In an emergency room patient with stroke symptoms, the initial diagnostic exam of choice would likely be:

    A. Carotid duplex
    B. CT
    C. MRI
    D. Cerebral angiography
    E. Radionucleotide study

190. Magnetic resonance angiography (MRA) functions by processing:

    A. X-ray frequency shifts from moving blood
    B. X-ray reflections from contrast material in the artery
    C. Isotope radiation using a scintillation camera
    D. Reflections from the hemoglobin in red blood cells
    E. Radiofrequency pulses created by tissue and blood flow

191. A pitfall of magnetic resonance angiography is:

    A. Patients with cardiac pacemakers cannot be studied.
    B. It requires the use of ionizing radiation.
    C. It tends to overestimate the degree of stenosis.
    D. It requires a high degree of patient cooperation.
    E. All but A
    F. All but B
    G. All but C

192. The endarterectomy procedure (removal of plaque from an artery):

    A. Is used only for carotid stenosis
    B. May be used for obstructed lower extremity arteries
    C. Is never used for infrarenal arteries
    D. Is a relatively recent surgical option
    E. Is the treatment of choice for obstructed renal arteries

193. Stenting procedures of the internal carotid artery:

    A. Are technically more demanding than stenting of coronary arteries
    B. Are technically less demanding than stenting of coronary arteries
    C. Are not currently being performed in the USA
    D. Carry a much lower risk of complications than carotid endarterectomy
    E. Are much less expensive than carotid endarterectomy

194. If a hypertensive patient has experienced multiple TIAs and has a 80% diameter stenosis of the internal carotid artery on the side referable to the symptoms:

   A. Carotid endarterectomy is probably recommended.
   B. Treatment of hypertension must be initiated immediately.
   C. Diabetes must be diagnosed.
   D. Renal artery stenosis should be treated first.
   E. Hypertension is not a significant risk factor in the development of carotid occlusive disease.

195. The NASCET trial indicated that the best treatment for carotid stenosis in the symptomatic patient is:

   A. Aspirin for stenosis greater than 70% in diameter
   B. Aspirin for stenosis greater than 70% in area
   C. Carotid endarterectomy for stenosis greater than 70% in diameter
   D. Carotid endarterectomy for stenosis greater than 70% in area
   E. Warfarin for stenosis less than 70% in diameter

196. The most common medical treatment of acute ischemic stroke consists of:

   A. Aspirin
   B. Dextran
   C. Heparin
   D. rtPA
   E. Dipyridamole

197. Hypertension is associated with hyperperfusion syndrome:

   A. Of the lower extremities
   B. Prior to a stroke
   C. After a stroke
   D. After carotid endarterectomy
   E. Prior to carotid endarterectomy

PART III

Venous Disease

Mechanisms of Venous Disease
Signs and Symptoms of Venous Disease
Testing and Treatment of Venous Disease

MECHANISMS OF VENOUS DISEASE

Risk factors

Acute venous thrombosis

Chronic deep venous obstruction

Chronic venous valvular insufficiency (primary, secondary)

Varicose veins

Congenital venous disorders

Pulmonary embolism

198. Which of these patients would LEAST likely be considered at high risk for deep venous thrombosis?

A. A 62-year-old woman with a fractured hip
B. A 36-year-old man with Hodgkin's disease
C. A 75-year-old woman admitted for transient ischemic attack
D. An 18-year-old male recovering from multiple injuries sustained in a motorcycle accident
E. A 72-year-old, overweight woman with congestive heart failure

199. The primary concern in patients with acute deep venous thrombosis is:

A. Damage to venous valves may occur.
B. Pulmonary embolism may occur.
C. Venous hypertension may occlude arterial inflow.
D. Extension of deep vein thrombus may occlude the superficial veins.
E. Deep venous thrombosis causes the patient severe pain.

200. Some causes of deep venous thrombosis may be:

A. Trauma
B. Hypercoagulability
C. Extrinsic compression upon deep veins
D. Lymphangiitis
E. All except D

201. The greatest pressure of venous hypertension in secondary varicose veins occurs:

    A. At rest
    B. During muscle contraction
    C. During muscle relaxation
    D. While standing quietly
    E. While sleeping

202. Select the factor least likely to contribute to deep venous thrombosis:

    A. Diabetes
    B. Pelvic mass
    C. Previous DVT
    D. Hip replacement surgery
    E. Pregnancy and delivery

203. Virchow's triad includes:

    A. Aging, cancer, and bed rest
    B. Stasis, increased thrombogenesis, and aging
    C. Stasis, aging, and venous injury
    D. Aging, hypercoagulability, and intimal injury
    E. Stasis, hypercoagulability, and intimal injury

204. Which is NOT a risk factor for DVT?

    A. Cancer
    B. Surgery
    C. Age
    D. Smoking
    E. Bed rest

205. What percentage of pulmonary emboli originates from lower extremity deep venous thrombosis?

    A. >90%
    B. 75%
    C. About 50%
    D. 25%
    E. 10–15%

206. The vascular technologist knows that chronic venous insufficiency and ulceration are:

    A. Chronic but controllable
    B. Curable and controllable
    C. Chronic and uncontrollable
    D. Uncontrollable only
    E. Always severely disabling

207. Lymphedema may be caused by all EXCEPT:

    A. Obesity
    B. Trauma or surgical excision of lymph pathways
    C. Infection
    D. Inflammation
    E. Radiation and chemotherapy

208. A varicose vein is most often:

    A. A dilatation of a perforating vein
    B. A dilatation of the small saphenous vein
    C. A jugular vein aneurysm
    D. A popliteal vein aneurysm
    E. A dilatation of the great saphenous vein or superficial tributary

209. Varices resulting from deep-venous valvular insufficiency and incompetent perforators are called:

    A. Primary varices
    B. Secondary varices
    C. Congenital varices
    D. Genicular veins
    E. Spider veins

210. A Baker's cyst is a collection of:

    A. Synovial fluid from the knee joint
    B. Red blood cells in a venous sinus
    C. Interstitial fluid along a fascial border
    D. Fibrous tissue just beneath the skin
    E. White cells and other debris along an infected graft

211. A thrombus is found in a gastrocnemius muscular vein approximately a third of the way down the calf from the knee. If this were to propagate proximally, it would next involve:

    A. The posterior tibial veins
    B. The anterior tibial veins
    C. The peroneal veins
    D. The popliteal vein
    E. The superficial veins

212. A thrombus is found in a soleal vein, a bit proximal to mid calf. If this were to propagate, it would next involve:

    A. The posterior tibial veins
    B. The anterior tibial veins
    C. The popliteal vein
    D. The posterior arch vein
    E. The great saphenous vein

213. Approximately what percentage of untreated calf-vein thrombosis is thought to propagate to a proximal level (i.e., popliteal or above)?

   A. 3–5%

   B. 15–20%

   C. 50–60%

   D. More than 90%

   E. All calf-vein thrombosis propagates at least to the popliteal level

214. One complication of deep venous recanalization is:

   A. Damage to venous valves, allowing reflux

   B. Embolization of thrombus

   C. Less prominent superficial veins

   D. Pain in the area of thrombus

   E. Thickening of toenails and loss of hair growth

SIGNS & SYMPTOMS OF VENOUS DISEASE

Acute venous disease

Chronic venous disease (skin changes, lymphedema, ulceration)

215. Two weeks after a fracture of the femur, a 33-year-old female is seen for swelling of the calf of the same leg. The preliminary diagnosis, prior to performance of any noninvasive testing, should include:

   A. Arteriovenous fistula

   B. Deep venous thrombosis

   C. Popliteal entrapment

   D. Two of the above

   E. All three

216. Symptoms of chronic venous insufficiency might result from all EXCEPT:

   A. Calf-vein thrombosis

   B. Popliteal vein thrombosis

   C. Superficial insufficiency

   D. Iliac vein thrombosis

   E. Gastrocnemius muscular thrombosis

217. Patients suspected of having venous disease may complain of pain that is:

   A. Only during the day

   B. Not constant

   C. Relieved by elevation

   D. Not relieved by elevation

   E. Mostly felt at night

218. Patients complaining of pain, swelling, and erythema of the lower extremity may have deep venous thrombosis, but the vascular technologist knows that diagnosing DVT by these symptoms alone is approximately:

    A. 20–25% accurate
    B. 46–62% accurate
    C. 75–80% accurate
    D. 85–90% accurate
    E. 95–100% accurate

219. Edema caused by deep venous thrombosis is characterized by:

    A. Swelling of the feet
    B. Swelling in the ankles and feet
    C. Swelling in the ankles, legs, and feet
    D. Swelling in the ankles and legs but not the feet
    E. Swelling in the groin

220. All of the following are causes of or risk factors for acute deep venous thrombosis EXCEPT:

    A. Trauma
    B. Extrinsic compression upon deep veins
    C. Hypercoagulability
    D. Arthritis
    E. Cancer

221. Complaints of chronic unilateral lower extremity swelling, aching, and a sense of heaviness most likely suggest:

    A. Cardiac/systemic origin
    B. Lipidemia
    C. Postphlebitic syndrome
    D. Primary varicose veins
    E. Venous ulceration

222. A patient with chronic venous insufficiency complains of sudden onset of edema and pain in the affected leg. This may be related to:

    A. Recurrence of acute deep venous thrombosis
    B. Elevated right-heart pressures
    C. Failure to wear surgical support stockings
    D. Lymphedema secondary to chronic venous occlusion
    E. It is probably not vein-related.

223. Pitting edema of both lower extremities is likely related to:

    A. Cardiac or systemic origin
    B. Deep venous thrombosis
    C. Primary varicose veins
    D. Secondary varicose veins
    E. Lipidemia

224. Insufficient veins have the following flow characteristics:

    A. Cephalad blood flow may be normal while the patient is quietly standing.

B. Caudal blood flow may be abnormal while the patient is quietly standing.

C. Venous pressure at the ankle in the supine patient does not differ from that of normal limbs.

D. Venous pressure at the ankle in the walking patient is markedly increased compared to that of normal limbs.

E. A, B, and C

F. B, C, and D

225. With exercise in patients with postphlebitic syndrome, which of the following is FALSE?

A. These patients usually have a small decrease in venous pressure that returns rapidly after ceasing exercise.

B. They usually have a quick decrease in venous pressure that takes a minute or two to return to pre-exercise levels.

C. They sometimes have an increase in venous pressure.

D. They may develop venous claudication.

E. Secondary varices may appear more prominent.

226. Patients with a swollen limb who have just returned from a country where filariasis is endemic may be suspected of having:

A. Deep venous thrombosis

B. Lymphedema

C. Renal failure

D. Klippel-Trenaunay syndrome

E. Lipidemia

227. A patient presents with bilateral lower extremity edema and nephrotic syndrome. Thrombus is suspected at which level?

A. IVC

B. Iliac veins

C. Femoropopliteal veins

D. Portal vein

E. This does not suggest thrombosis.

228. Lower extremity ulcers are overwhelmingly the result of:

A. Arterial disease

B. Venous disease

C. Lymphatic disease

D. Cardiac disease and chronic right-heart congestion

E. Hyperlipidemia

229. Normally, venous flow in the calf is from the superficial to the deep veins through perforating veins. However, this flow might be reversed when:

    A. There is superficial vein phlebitis.
    B. The individual is ambulatory.
    C. There are varicosities.
    D. Deep venous obstruction is present.
    E. Congestive heart failure is present.

230. A patient presents with acute pronounced bright red discoloration and edema of the skin along the anterior calf. The most likely diagnosis is:

    A. Superficial thrombophlebitis
    B. Deep vein thrombosis
    C. Cellulitis
    D. Chronic venous insufficiency
    E. Incompetent perforating veins

231. A patient with a pulmonary embolus might have any of these EXCEPT:

    A. Chest pain
    B. Reduced arterial blood gasses
    C. Diaphoresis
    D. Shortness of breath
    E. Rest pain

232. Typical findings of skin discoloration in a patient with chronic venous insufficiency are:

    A. Cyanotic (bluish) color in toes and feet
    B. Bright red, mottled skin on anterolateral calf and thigh
    C. Pallor on elevation, rubor on dependency of limb
    D. Rusty brown color at ankles and calves
    E. Bruised-appearing, purple areas on dorsum of feet

233. A condition that presents as a severely swollen, blue, cool lower extremity is called:

    A. Stasis dermatitis
    B. Phlegmasia alba dolens
    C. Phlegmasia cerulea dolens
    D. Cellulitis
    E. Lymphedema

234. The clinical examination for deep venous thrombosis is:

    A. Specific and sensitive
    B. Not specific but sensitive
    C. Specific but not sensitive
    D. Neither specific nor sensitive
    E. None of the above

235. Which of the following are NOT associated with chronic venous disease?

    A. Pigmentation
    B. Brawny edema
    C. Subcutaneous fibrosis
    D. Cutaneous atrophy
    E. Thickening of toenails

236. Which of the following is TRUE regarding chronic venous ulceration?

    A. Lesions are frequently found on the foot.
    B. Pain is severe and is relieved by dependency.
    C. Lesions are usually found on the lower third of the leg around the medial aspect of the ankle.
    D. Lesions do not ooze blood when manipulated.
    E. Granulation tissue is not produced during healing.

237. Some time after being hit by a car, a patient has severe pain in the anterior aspect of the right knee and massive left lower extremity edema. The patient most likely has:

    A. Bilateral superficial venous thrombosis
    B. Localized right popliteal deep venous thrombosis
    C. Localized left popliteal deep venous thrombosis
    D. Extensive left femoropopliteal deep venous thrombosis
    E. Extensive right femoropopliteal deep venous thrombosis

238. An elderly patient who presents with localized pain at mid calf has an ultrasound exam that reveals a nonocclusive thrombus of the femoral vein. The calf pain became excruciating after administration of heparin. A second ultrasound exam demonstrates:

    A. Progression of deep venous thrombosis to the popliteal and calf veins
    B. Nonocclusive thrombus at the superficial femoral
    C. A popliteal aneurysm
    D. A hypoechoic mass in the shape of an egg at mid calf, thought to be a hematoma
    E. A Baker's cyst in the popliteal fossa

239. A patient presents with a unilateral chronic swollen leg and a previous diagnosis of deep venous thrombosis 3 years earlier. The most likely finding would be:

    A. The popliteal vein is thrombosed.
    B. The popliteal vein is patent and the valves competent.
    C. The popliteal vein is patent and the valves are incompetent.
    D. Venography is necessary to distinguish old from new thrombus.
    E. The patient has congestive heart failure.

240. Chronic deep venous obstruction will increase:

    A. Venous flow
    B. Arterial inflow
    C. Resting supine venous pressure
    D. Ambulatory venous pressure
    E. Ambulatory residual venous volume

241. Brawny skin changes at the ankle most likely represent:

    A. Acute valvular insufficiency
    B. Acute deep venous thrombosis
    C. Chronic venous insufficiency
    D. Acute arterial ischemia
    E. Chronic arterial ischemia

242. Select the best statement regarding comparison of venous and arterial ulcers:

    A. Venous ulcers are usually not painful and are located on the foot.
    B. Venous ulcers are usually not painful and are located cephalad to the foot.
    C. Venous ulcers are usually painful and are located cephalad to the foot.
    D. Venous ulcers are associated with decreased arterial pulses.
    E. Arterial ulcers are treated with Unna boots.

243. Signs that a general practitioner may use in an attempt to diagnose deep venous thrombosis include all of the following EXCEPT:

    A. Passive dorsiflexion of foot (Homans' sign)
    B. Anteroposterior calf compression (Bancroft's sign)
    C. Inflating a sphygmomanometer to 80 mmHg on calf (Lowenberg's sign)
    D. Tourniquet test
    E. Physical findings of edema

244. A common physical finding in pulmonary embolism is:

    A. Apnea
    B. Bradycardia
    C. Thrombocytopenia
    D. Bradypenia
    E. Tachypnea

245. All of the following may be found in the clinical presentation of pulmonary embolism EXCEPT:

    A. Chest pain
    B. Dyspnea
    C. Pleural effusion
    D. Positive lower extremity venous ultrasound
    E. Tachypnea

TESTING & TREATMENT OF VENOUS DISEASE

Noninvasive testing (patient positioning, technique, interpretation, capabilities, limitations)

Acute venous thrombosis (duplex imaging and continuous-wave Doppler)

Chronic venous insufficiency or obstruction (duplex imaging, reflux plethysmography)

Venography

Treatment

246. Which of these is NOT true about superficial thrombophlebitis in the leg?

    A. It is usually attributed to a thrombosed saphenous vein.
    B. It can best be diagnosed by photoplethysmography.
    C. It may result in significant incapacitation for the patient.
    D. It usually responds to ambulation, warm soaks, and aspirin.
    E. It is frequently recurrent.

247. The most reliable method for establishing the diagnosis of pulmonary embolism is:

    A. Duplex ultrasound
    B. Pulmonary angiography
    C. V/Q scan
    D. Chest x-ray
    E. ECG

248. Doppler examination alone, without B-mode, is unlikely to detect the presence of venous thrombosis in:

    A. The femoral vein
    B. The subclavian vein
    C. A peroneal vein
    D. The popliteal vein
    E. The common femoral vein

249. A patient is seated with legs dangling and a photoplethysmograph sensor placed just above the medial malleolus. After dorsiflexion of the foot five times, this tracing is made. The tracing is consistent with:

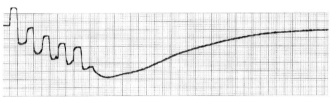

    A. Superficial venous insufficiency
    B. Calf vein obstruction
    C. Deep venous insufficiency
    D. Essentially normal venous refilling
    E. Superficial vein incompetence

250. A 46-year-old man comes to the vascular laboratory with calf and ankle edema, mild discomfort in the calf, and a soft mass behind the knee. Continuous-wave Doppler studies are negative except for some continuous flow over the popliteal vein. An additional test that might be useful is:

    A. Venous reflux plethysmography
    B. Venous outflow
    C. Spectral analysis
    D. Ultrasound imaging

E. Photoplethysmography

251. In continuous-wave Doppler reflux testing, a normal result is:

    A. Cessation of flow with proximal compression, resuming on release
    B. Cessation of flow with distal compression, remaining absent on release
    C. Augmentation of flow with proximal compression, ceasing with release
    D. Augmentation of flow with distal compression, continuing with release
    E. Augmentation of flow with Valsalva maneuver

252. The test for venous incompetence that uses tourniquets and alterations of patient position is called:

    A. Photoplethysmography
    B. The Trendelenburg test
    C. The Hunter's canal test
    D. The Ferris and Kistener test
    E. Light reflection rheography test

253. A continuous-wave Doppler examination of the lower extremities, performed to diagnose deep vein thrombophlebitis, revealed augmentation upon compression proximal to the probe at all standard levels studied. The diagnosis is:

    A. Femoral deep venous thrombosis
    B. Femoropopliteal deep venous thrombosis
    C. Femoropopliteal valvular insufficiency
    D. Femoropopliteal and posterior tibial valvular insufficiency
    E. Femoropopliteal and posterior tibial deep venous thrombosis

254. Venous refilling time by photoplethysmography was 10 seconds without a tourniquet applied and 25 seconds with a tourniquet applied to the lower thigh. The diagnosis is:

    A. Deep and superficial valvular insufficiency
    B. Deep valvular insufficiency
    C. Superficial valvular insufficiency
    D. Superficial venous thrombosis
    E. Deep venous thrombosis

255. The examiner listens with CW Doppler to the femoral vein at mid thigh and performs a calf compression. The compression maneuver augments the signal. This finding suggests:

    A. Deep vein thrombosis at the iliac level
    B. Deep vein thrombosis at the femoral level
    C. Deep vein thrombosis in calf veins
    D. Valvular incompetence
    E. This is a normal finding.

256. During a duplex venous exam, which of the following findings is the least likely to be associated with acute deep venous thrombosis?

    A. Continuous venous flow
    B. Stationary echoes within the vein

C. Homogeneous intraluminal echoes

D. Venous reflux

E. Enlarged incompressible vein

257. Of the following techniques, which would be the least effective in detecting significant DVT?

   A. Photoplethysmography
   B. Duplex ultrasound
   C. Impedance plethysmography
   D. Pneumoplethysmography
   E. Strain-gauge plethysmography

258. Most often, the settings for venous color flow imaging of the lower extremities:

   A. Are the same as those for peripheral arterial studies
   B. Are the same as those for abdominal arterial scanning
   C. Are the same as those for carotid scanning
   D. Are the same as those for abdominal venous scanning
   E. Are different from any of the above

259. When performing lower extremity venous Doppler assessment in normal patients, cephalad flow diminishes:

   A. During Valsalva maneuver
   B. During inspiration
   C. During expiration
   D. During proximal compression
   E. All but C

260. On CW Doppler assessment, a patient with a swollen left leg has loud, continuous flow signals from the left great saphenous vein. The asymptomatic leg has nonspontaneous flow in the right great saphenous vein, which augments with distal compression. These findings are consistent with:

   A. Normal venous flow
   B. Right-leg DVT
   C. Left-leg DVT
   D. Bilateral DVT
   E. These findings are not helpful diagnostically.

261. The Valsalva maneuver:

   A. Increases pressure in the thoracic cavity, decreases pressure in the abdominal cavity
   B. Decreases pressure in the thoracic cavity, increases pressure in the abdominal cavity
   C. Slows down or stops venous flow everywhere in the body
   D. Increases venous flow everywhere in the body
   E. Affects arterial, not venous, flow

262. Which of the following is NOT one of the commonly assessed characteristics of CW venous Doppler?

A. Spontaneity
B. Gaiety
C. Augmentation
D. Competence
E. Phasicity

263. A patient presents with a swollen right lower extremity. Duplex imaging demonstrates patency of the femoral, popliteal, and calf veins. However, Doppler at the common femoral level on the right is continuous, not changing with respiration, while Doppler of the left common femoral vein is phasic. These findings might suggest:

A. Thrombosis of the profunda femoris vein
B. Right iliac thrombosis
C. Left iliac thrombosis
D. Vena cava thrombosis
E. This is not a diagnostically useful finding.

264. The optimal patient position for imaging of the lower extremity veins is:

A. Semi-Fowler's position
B. Trendelenburg's position
C. Reverse Trendelenburg's position
D. Supine, leg elevated
E. Answers A and C

265. Demonstration of vein-wall coaptation in the extremities is best performed:

A. In a longitudinal plane with the color flow documenting cephalad flow
B. In a longitudinal plane without color flow
C. In a transverse plane with the color flow documenting patency
D. In a transverse plane without color flow
E. Coaptation is seldom diagnostic in duplex imaging.

266. The examiner uses color flow to assess for competence at the common femoral vein level. With Valsalva maneuver, there is red flow lasting approximately half a second, then blue flow on release of Valsalva.

A. This finding is within normal limits.
B. This finding is equivocal for significant valvular incompetence.
C. This finding confirms significant valvular incompetence.
D. This finding suggests AV fistula.
E. This finding confirms deep vein thrombosis.

267. Signs on duplex venous imaging of acute rather than chronic deep vein thrombosis include all EXCEPT:

A. Bright intraluminal echoes
B. Distended vein
C. Dark intraluminal echoes
D. Slightly compressible (spongy) character to thrombus
E. Presence of a "tail" suggesting poor adherence to wall

268. Limitations of handheld CW Doppler venous assessment include all EXCEPT:

    A. There may be bifid superficial femoral or popliteal veins.
    B. Non-occluding thrombus may not be detected.
    C. A collateral vein may be mistaken for the vein of intended assessment.
    D. Exact extent cannot be determined for follow-up studies.
    E. Valvular incompetence cannot be assessed with CW Doppler.

269. The examiner scans the femoral veins and notes a very small venous lumen, with bright, thickened venous walls along most of the thigh. These findings suggest:

    A. Acute DVT
    B. AV fistula
    C. Chronic thrombosis
    D. Congenitally hypoplastic veins
    E. Arterial, not venous, insufficiency.

270. Thrombosis that appears on duplex scan to be dark, homogeneous in character, and poorly attached to the venous wall suggests:

    A. Old, partially recanalized thrombosis
    B. Acute thrombosis
    C. Artifactual echoes
    D. Acoustic "doubling" of the image due to the presence of a strong interface
    E. A nondiagnostic image

271. The examiner scans a patient with pain and swelling in the calf. A large, dark area is noted in the medial popliteal space, and no vascular communication to it is found. This most likely represents:

    A. Popliteal aneurysm
    B. Cystic adventitial degeneration
    C. Cellulitis
    D. Necrosis
    E. Baker's cyst

272. In a reflux study, the examiner images the popliteal vein and notes that the venous color flow display lights up blue with calf compression, then red for 2–3 seconds on release.

    A. This is within normal limits.
    B. This confirms deep venous thrombosis.
    C. This is normal, but the color flow assignment is reversed.
    D. This suggests venous reflux.
    E. This is nondiagnostic without probe compression to make the walls coapt.

273. The area in the lower extremity where it is usually most difficult to bring about vein-wall coaptation with probe compression is:

    A. The saphenofemoral junction
    B. The mid thigh
    C. The distal thigh

  D. The popliteal space
  E. The mid calf

274. A long, brightly-echogenic streak is noted in the common femoral vein, which is otherwise patent and compressible. It moves with probe compression and appears to move with venous flow. This is most likely:

  A. An artifact due to excessive imaging gain and reverberation
  B. A valve leaflet
  C. A remnant of recanalized old DVT
  D. Acute thrombosis in evolution
  E. Embolic material from an aneurysmal popliteal vein

275. Pulsatile lower extremity venous Doppler signals would be associated with:

  A. Deep vein thrombosis
  B. Acute arterial occlusion
  C. Congestive heart failure
  D. Severe superficial vein valvular insufficiency
  E. CVA

276. Continuous-wave Doppler assessment of the posterior tibial level reveals nonspontaneous flow that augments with foot compression. This finding:

  A. Confirms deep vein thrombosis
  B. Is within normal limits in a cold patient
  C. Is within normal limits in a warm patient
  D. Confirms valvular incompetence proximally
  E. Suggests CHF

277. The following tracing is taken from a patient with chronic ankle and calf edema. The PPG sensor is placed slightly proximal to the medial malleolus, and the patient dorsiflexes five times, then relaxes. The tracing:

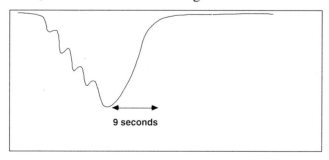

9 seconds

  A. Suggests significant valvular incompetence
  B. Is within normal limits
  C. Is equivocal
  D. Suggests not venous but arterial insufficiency
  E. Suggests acute deep vein thrombosis

278. The test on the aforementioned patient is repeated, this time with a tourniquet around the leg just below the knee. There is no appreciable change in the tracing. This finding:

A. Suggests superficial valvular incompetence only
B. Suggests deep venous valvular incompetence
C. Is equivocal
D. Rules out venous causes for the edema
E. Using a tourniquet is not part of the usual PPG reflux protocol.

279. Descending venography is performed to diagnose:

A. Femoral venous thrombosis
B. Valvular insufficiency
C. Popliteal venous thrombosis
D. Superficial venous thrombosis
E. Inferior vena cava valvular insufficiency

280. Contrast venography is:

A. Dangerous
B. Not sensitive
C. Invasive
D. Not specific
E. Not indicated when DVT is clinically suspected

281. The venous puncture for introducing contrast in venography to assess for deep venous thrombosis is done at what level?

A. Common femoral vein
B. Great saphenous vein just distal to the saphenofemoral junction
C. Popliteal vein
D. Dorsal vein on the foot
E. Internal jugular vein, to avoid influencing lower extremity hemodynamics

282. The venous puncture for introducing contrast in venography to assess for valvular insufficiency is done at what level?

A. Common femoral vein
B. Contrast is not used for insufficiency testing
C. Popliteal vein
D. Dorsal vein on the foot
E. Internal jugular vein, to avoid influencing lower extremity hemodynamics

283. The patient position for venography is:

    A. Supine, leg elevated
    B. Trendelenburg's position
    C. Seated, legs dependent
    D. On an exam table tilted 60 degrees upright
    E. Standing on floor, with weight on the nonsymptomatic leg

284. Potential complications of venography include all EXCEPT:

    A. Allergic reaction to contrast
    B. Toxicity to kidneys
    C. Arteriovenous fistula
    D. Iatrogenic CVA
    E. Thrombophlebitis

285. Acute deep venous thrombosis is commonly indicated in venography as:

    A. Area of increased contrast taken up by the thrombus
    B. Area of no contrast, often with "railroad track" lines along walls
    C. Area of intermittently reduced contrast, commonly referred to as a "string of pearls"
    D. Primarily well-developed collaterals around the knee and groin
    E. Complete blockage of the superficial veins and perforators

286. The "gold standard" test for pulmonary embolus, though it carries its own risk for compromised patients, is:

    A. Ascending venography
    B. Descending venography
    C. V/Q scan
    D. Pulmonary angiography
    E. IVC opacification testing

287. A radioisotope test for pulmonary embolism that involves both breathing and injection of the isotope, and is usually reported in "high, medium, or low probability" of pulmonary embolus, is called:

    A. IVC opacification testing
    B. V/Q scan
    C. Swan-Ganz catheterization
    D. Arterial blood gasses
    E. Pulmonary function testing

288. The drug heparin:

    A. Affects the prothrombin time
    B. Directly attacks formed thrombi
    C. Is reversed by administration of vitamin K
    D. Is safe
    E. Can cause thrombocytopenia

289. Chronic venous insufficiency frequently leads to ulceration. The vascular technologist knows that the patient can help prevent ulceration by:

    A. Elevating the legs above heart level more than 4 times a day for 20 minutes
    B. Using support stockings when ambulatory
    C. A and B above
    D. Chelation therapy
    E. Taking aspirin

290. The following are all possible complications of heparin EXCEPT:

    A. Thrombocytopenia
    B. Formation of antiplatelet antibody
    C. Decreased activated partial thromboplastin time
    D. Intraabdominal bleeding
    E. Increased bruising

291. After the initial dose of heparin, the current standard of treatment for deep venous thrombosis consists of placing the patient on the following medication for 3 or more months:

    A. Streptokinase
    B. Urokinase
    C. Tissue plasminogen activator
    D. Vitamin K
    E. Sodium warfarin

292. Commonly performed methods of vena cava interruption for recurrent pulmonary embolism include all of the following EXCEPT:

    A. The bird's nest filter
    B. The Greenfield umbrella filter
    C. The nitinol filter
    D. The Vena Tech filter
    E. The Jones wire arch

293. Possible complications of vena cava interruption for recurrent pulmonary embolism include all of the following EXCEPT:

    A. Diminished cardiac output
    B. Edema
    C. Leg ulcers
    D. Venous claudication
    E. Night cramps

294. The agent of choice in the initial management of pulmonary embolism is:

    A. Heparin
    B. Streptokinase
    C. Urokinase
    D. Coumadin
    E. Tissue plasminogen activator

PART IV

Peripheral Arterial Disease

Mechanisms of Peripheral Arterial Disease
Signs and Symptoms of Peripheral Arterial Disease
Testing and Treatment of Peripheral Arterial Disease

MECHANISMS OF PERIPHERAL ARTERIAL DISEASE

Risk factors

Atherosclerosis

Embolism

Aneurysm

Nonatherosclerotic lesions

295. The etiology of arterial aneurysms includes all of the following EXCEPT:

   A. Syphilitic
   B. Degenerative
   C. Inflammatory
   D. Congenital
   E. Saccular

296. More than 90% of infrarenal abdominal aneurysms are of:

   A. Traumatic origin
   B. Degenerative origin
   C. Anastomotic origin
   D. Infectious origin
   E. Syphilitic origin

297. A condition that causes nonatherosclerotic narrowing of brachiocephalic arteries in overwhelmingly female patients is called:

   A. Compartment syndrome
   B. Raynaud's syndrome
   C. Takayasu's arteritis
   D. Fibromuscular dysplasia
   E. Buerger's disease

298. The most common source of lower or upper extremity peripheral arterial embolus is:

   A. Ulcerated plaque

B. The heart

C. Aneurysms

D. Arterial dissections and atherosclerosis

E. Small vessel arteriosclerosis

299. Aneurysms are most often caused by:

A. Trauma

B. Systemic infection

C. Pregnancy

D. Congenital arterial wall weakness

E. Bifurcated laminar flow

300. An occlusive disease of medium and small arteries in the distal upper and lower limbs of primarily young male heavy smokers is:

A. Raynaud's syndrome

B. Thromboangiitis obliterans

C. Atherosclerosis obliterans

D. Periarteritis nodosa

E. Hyperlipoproteinemia

301. A condition which might result from reperfusion edema following bypass surgery, causing ischemia due to compression, and which might call for treatment by fasciotomy, is called:

A. Marfan's syndrome

B. Compartment syndrome

C. Raynaud's syndrome

D. Thoracic outlet syndrome

E. China syndrome

302. The combination of neuropathy and peripherally distributed atherosclerosis makes the diabetic patient especially vulnerable to:

A. Aortoiliac disease

B. Popliteal entrapment syndrome

C. Foot lesions

D. Abdominal aortic aneurysms

E. Renal artery lesions

303. The chance of a patient dying from a rupture of an abdominal aortic aneurysm averages:

A. 25%

B. 35%

C. 45%

D. 55%

E. 80%

304. Which of the following statements is FALSE regarding smoking?

    A. It accelerates the onset and progression of atherosclerosis.
    B. It increases the oxygen-carrying capacity of blood.
    C. Cigarette smoke contains nearly 5,000 chemicals.
    D. It causes swelling of endothelial cells.
    E. It increases platelet aggregation and adherence.

305. In the lower extremity circulation, the most common site of atherosclerosis is:

    A. The arterial segment beginning at the popliteal artery
    B. The arterial segment beginning in Hunter's canal
    C. The arterial segment at the iliac bifurcation
    D. The proximal tibial vessels
    E. The arterial segment at the popliteal trifurcations

306. Which of the following statements about popliteal aneurysms is TRUE?

    A. They pose a significant risk to the patient due to rupture.
    B. They can cause symptoms by compressing contiguous structures.
    C. They pose a significant risk of limb loss due to embolism or occlusion.
    D. They are found bilaterally in > 10% of cases where they exist.
    E. Claudication is a rare symptom.
    F. A and D
    G. B, C, and D

307. Which of the following statements regarding abdominal aortic aneurysms is FALSE?

    A. AAAs are usually infrarenal.
    B. Computerized tomography and MRI are common modalities for the diagnosis of AAA.
    C. Ultrasound imaging is the most frequently used modality for diagnosis of AAA.
    D. Abdominal aneurysms pose a significant risk of rupture if > 6 cm in diameter.
    E. Most prerupture AAAs are discovered because of abdominal symptoms or distal emboli.

308. The risk of claudication in diabetic patients is:

    A. Equal to the risk in the general population.
    B. Greater than 4 times the risk in the general population.
    C. Close to 10% of the risk in the general population.
    D. Lower than that in the general population.
    E. Claudication is not an ischemic symptom for diabetics.

309. Select the entity that is NOT a risk factor in peripheral arterial occlusive disease:

    A. Hypolipidemia
    B. Smoking
    C. Hypertension
    D. Diabetes
    E. Hyperlipidemia

SIGNS & SYMPTOMS OF PERIPHERAL ARTERIAL DISEASE

Chronic peripheral arterial disease (claudication, rest pain, tissue loss)

Acute peripheral arterial occlusion (thrombosis, emboli)

Vasospastic disorders

Physical examination (skin changes, pulse palpation, auscultation)

310. The vascular disease that presents as back, abdominal, or flank pain is:

    A. Intracranial arterial disease
    B. Abdominal aortic aneurysm
    C. Iliofemoral occlusive disease
    D. Superior mesenteric stenosis
    E. Renal artery stenosis

311. Takayasu's arteritis is most often found in:

    A. Young men
    B. Middle-aged men
    C. Elderly men
    D. Young women
    E. Elderly women

312. Common signs of advanced arterial insufficiency of the lower extremity include which of the following?

    A. Loss of hair growth over the dorsum of the toes and feet
    B. Thickening of the toenails
    C. Dermatitis with skin pigmentation
    D. Dependent rubor
    E. A, B, and D

313. The term *cyanosis* describes:

    A. Blue color of tissue due to ischemia
    B. Red color of tissue due to hyperemia
    C. Pale skin due to ischemia
    D. Thickening of toenails due to chronic ischemia
    E. Loss of hair growth due to chronic ischemia

314. Match the following symptoms and signs with the likely cause. (*Tip:* Start with the most obvious and work your way in.)

    A. Bruit   1. Aortoiliac + SFA occlusion
    B. Absent pulse   2. Deep venous thrombosis
    C. Foot rubor   3. Subclavian artery occlusion (acute)
    D. Right sided weakness   4. Left carotid artery occlusion
    E. Edema   5. Iliac artery stenosis

315. A common evaluation for advanced lower extremity ischemia involves raising the supine patient's leg and then having the patient sit and dangle the leg. A positive result is described as:

    A. Elevation pallor, dependent rubor
    B. Elevation rubor, dependent pallor
    C. Elevation paresthesia, dependent pain
    D. Elevation rubor, dependent cyanosis
    E. Elevation pallor, dependent cyanosis

316. Patients presenting with symptoms of claudication complain of:

    A. Nocturnal muscle cramps
    B. Cramping pain in the calf, thigh, or buttocks with exercise and relieved by rest
    C. Numbing weakness in the legs while standing
    D. Pain in hips or knees not relieved by rest
    E. Cramping pain in the calf, thigh, or buttocks with exercise not relieved by rest

317. Patients presenting with a diagnosis of ischemic rest pain may complain of:

    A. Foot pain at night which occurs on an irregular basis
    B. Tingling in the foot which is relieved by elevation
    C. Foot pain while in a horizontal position, relieved by standing or dangling the foot in a dependent position
    D. A numbing weakness produced by standing
    E. Pain in feet with walking which is relieved by rest

318. Patients found to have ulcerating lesions or gangrene may have which of the following diseases?

    A. Arterial insufficiency
    B. Neuropathy
    C. Vasospasm
    D. Venous disease
    E. All of the above

319. The most common presenting symptoms in acute arterial occlusion include all EXCEPT:

    A. Paralysis
    B. Pulselessness
    C. Pallor
    D. Paresthesias
    E. Pedal ulcer

320. Patients with advanced peripheral arterial vascular occlusive disease exhibit which of the following skin changes?

    A. Shiny, scaly skin
    B. Dependent rubor
    C. Pallor on elevation
    D. Stasis pigmentation
    E. All except D

321. A 54-year-old male relates a history of calf and thigh pain, the right worse than the left. This pain resolves upon sitting down. The pain usually starts after the first few steps of walking, but does not limit the patient's ability to walk three blocks. Since he never walks more than this distance, he cannot relate that he would have to stop at a greater distance. Some days the pain is quite mild. The etiology of these symptoms can be:

   A. Abdominal aortic disease
   B. Bilateral iliac artery disease
   C. Bilateral superficial femoral and profunda disease
   D. A, B, and C are potential etiologies
   E. These symptoms are not typical of vascular disease

322. A diabetic patient with redness of the skin in the foot and toe probably has:

   A. An infection
   B. Emboli
   C. Increased sympathetic tone
   D. Low central temperature
   E. Popliteal aneurysm

323. A pulsatile mass in the groin after catheterization of a cardiac patient most likely will be:

   A. A femoral artery aneurysm
   B. A hematoma
   C. A pseudoaneurysm of the femoral artery
   D. A false aneurysm of the femoral vein
   E. An arteriovenous fistula

324. Early atherosclerosis of the lower extremities will be associated with:

   A. Rest pain
   B. Blue toe
   C. Claudication
   D. Pregangrene
   E. Swelling

325. Which sign or symptom is least likely to be associated with arterial embolization?

   A. Blue toe
   B. TIA
   C. Popliteal aneurysm
   D. Amaurosis fugax
   E. Progressive claudication

326. Rest pain is characterized by:

   A. Upper calf pain
   B. Pain at night in the forefoot or foot that may go away with leg dependency
   C. Pain while walking that goes away with rest
   D. Upper calf pain that goes away with leg dependency
   E. Any calf pain that goes away with leg dependency

327. The symptom or sign most likely NOT associated with acute arterial occlusion is:

    A. Blue toe
    B. Pain of sudden onset
    C. Pale or white extremity
    D. Claudication
    E. Paresthesia

328. Ischemic ulcers (lesions) are:

    A. Completely painless but bleed with manipulation and are located over pressure points or calluses.
    B. Very painful and commonly located distally over the dorsum of the foot.
    C. Only mildly painful and relieved by elevation.
    D. Very painful and are usually located around the malleolus.
    E. Caused by pathogenic organisms.

329. Common sites for auscultation of bruits in the lower extremity circulation include all EXCEPT:

    A. Abdomen
    B. Groin
    C. Popliteal space
    D. Dorsum of foot
    E. All are common auscultatory sites

330. A vibration noted while palpating pulses is called:

    A. A buzz
    B. A bruit
    C. A scintillation
    D. A pulse
    E. A thrill

331. Rubor is defined as:

    A. Abnormal stiffness of digits
    B. Small, purple areas of discoloration on the dorsum of the foot
    C. Thickened, wrinkled skin
    D. Red skin color
    E. Slackening of the muscles of the ischemic foot

332. Ulcers due to arterial insufficiency are found most often:

    A. Behind the knee
    B. In the gaiter area, near the medial malleolus
    C. On toes and distal foot
    D. Over the lesion, usually along Hunter's canal
    E. Mid calf

333. Delayed return of the capillary blush after pressure on the pulp of the digit is a sign of:

A. Thoracic outlet syndrome
B. Venous occlusive disease
C. Advanced ischemia
D. Hyperlipidemia
E. Hypercholesterolemia

334. Signs of advanced ischemia in the lower extremity include all of the following EXCEPT:

    A. Slow venous filling after dropping the elevated extremity into a dependent position
    B. Pallor on elevation
    C. Rubor on dependency
    D. Pitting edema
    E. Ulceration at the dorsum of the foot

335. Pulse sites commonly palpated in the lower extremities include all EXCEPT:

    A. Common femoral
    B. Popliteal
    C. Posterior tibial
    D. Anterior tibial
    E. Peroneal

336. The absence of a bruit at the common femoral level:

    A. Rules out significant stenosis at that level
    B. Cannot rule out significant stenosis at that level
    C. Suggests stenosis distal to that level
    D. Suggests total occlusion at that level
    E. Suggests stenosis proximal to that level

337. Auscultation of the abdomen, aortoiliac, and common femoral areas is important because:

    A. Absence of a bruit suggests absence of arterial disease.
    B. Presence of a bruit may be the first indication of arterial disease.
    C. Abdominal bruits are significant because they are usually radiating from the aortic arch.
    D. Only significant stenosis can cause bruits.
    E. B, C, and D.

338. The symptoms of anterior tibial compartment syndrome are:

    A. Swelling and/or palpable tenderness over a muscle compartment
    B. Sensory deficit or paresthesias
    C. Pain on passive stretch of the muscles in the compartment
    D. Weakness of the muscles in the compartment
    E. All of the above

339. Unilateral claudication in the calf and foot of a young individual suggests:

    A. Popliteal artery entrapment
    B. Anterior tibial compartment syndrome
    C. "Restless" leg syndrome

D. Lumbar disc disease

E. Arteriosclerosis

340. A patient complains of digital pallor or cyanosis induced by cold exposure or emotional stimuli. These symptoms are characteristic of:

A. Arterial embolism to the digits

B. Raynaud's phenomenon

C. Thoracic outlet syndrome

D. Carpal tunnel syndrome

E. Klippel-Trenaunay-Weber syndrome

TESTING AND TREATMENT OF PERIPHERAL ARTERIAL DISEASE

Noninvasive testing (patient positioning, technique, interpretation, capabilities, limitations)

Miscellaneous diagnostic tests (methods, interpretation, limitations)

Arteriography

MR Angiography

CT

Treatment of peripheral arterial disease (medical, endovascular, surgical)

Physical examination (skin changes, pulse palpation, auscultation)

341. The pulsatility index is defined as:

A. Peak systolic velocity divided by end diastolic velocity.

B. Peak systolic velocity minus end diastolic velocity divided by systolic velocity.

C. Peak systolic velocity minus mean velocity divided by systolic velocity.

D. Peak systolic to peak end diastolic velocity divided by mean velocity.

E. Peak systolic velocity at the internal carotid artery divided by peak systolic velocity at the common carotid artery.

342. Which one of the following is always TRUE of patients who suffer from intermittent claudication?

A. Peripheral blood flow is reduced at rest.

B. There is pressure drop distal to the obstructed segment after exercise.

C. No increase in blood flow occurs through the affected segment during exercise.

D. Marked peripheral vasoconstriction occurs in response to exercise.

E. There is always a pressure drop distal to the obstructed segment at rest.

343. Which one of the following conditions will cause an increase in the pulse amplitude of the arterial pressure wave?

A. An increase in peripheral resistance

B. A decrease in left ventricular function

C. Vasodilation secondary to heating

D. Young age

E. Mild atherosclerosis

344. Which one of the following changes occurs in the peripheral blood flow of limbs with obstructive arterial disease in response to laboratory-induced ischemia (reactive hyperemia procedure) or exercise?

   A. Flow increases more in obstructed limbs than in limbs with no obstruction.
   B. Hyperemia is prolonged in obstructed limbs in comparison to limbs with no obstruction.
   C. Flow decreases in order to redistribute blood volume to the central circulation.
   D. Cardiac output is reduced.
   E. Peripheral resistance is increased due to muscle contraction.

345. Ankle/arm indices in claudicating patients are usually:

   A. Not a useful test for this condition
   B. In the range of 1.0–1.5
   C. In the range of 0.5–0.9
   D. In the range of 0.1–0.3
   E. Artificially elevated

346. The ankle/arm index is obtained by dividing the:

   A. Higher of the two brachial pressures by ankle pressure
   B. Lower of the two brachial pressures by ankle pressure
   C. Ankle pressure by the lower brachial pressure
   D. Ankle pressure by the higher brachial pressure
   E. Ankle pressure by the average of the two brachial pressures

347. A velocity obtained in the mid superficial femoral artery is 225 cm/sec, while a measurement just proximal to this site gives 90 cm/sec. This suggests:

   A. SFA aneurysm
   B. Mild SFA stenosis
   C. SFA occlusion
   D. >50% SFA stenosis
   E. >80% SFA stenosis

348. The right high-thigh pressure measurement is 108 mmHg, while the left high-thigh is 142 mmHg. Brachial pressure is 122 mmHg. Of the following, this most likely suggests:

   A. Right femoral artery obstruction
   B. Left femoral artery obstruction
   C. Aortoiliac obstruction
   D. Left iliac artery obstruction
   E. Right popliteal artery obstruction

349. The key technology in arterial pneumoplethysmography is:

   A. Two pairs of electrode bands monitoring impedance changes in a limb segment
   B. Two photocells monitoring subcutaneous color changes
   C. A pressure transducer monitoring cuff pressure over a limb

    D. A silastic tube filled with mercury that changes resistance with changes of limb circumference

    E. A large air cuff enclosing the entire calf

350. When assessing a digital artery with Doppler, patency of the palmar arch can be determined by:

    A. Compressing the brachial artery while listening for changes in the digital artery signal

    B. Compressing the radial artery while listening for changes in the digital artery signal

    C. Compressing the ulnar artery while listening for changes in the digital artery signal

    D. Alternately compressing the radial and ulnar arteries while listening for changes in the digital artery signal

    E. Inflating a digital cuff to suprasystolic pressure

351. Assessment of palmar arch patency is useful:

    A. Before placement of an arteriovenous arm shunt

    B. When evaluating a patient with suspected subclavian steal

    C. To evaluate blood flow to the digital arteries

    D. A and B

    E. A and C

352. An analog Doppler waveform of the subclavian or axillary artery in a normal individual would typically resemble:

    A. A common carotid artery waveform

    B. A vertebral artery waveform

    C. A common femoral or superficial femoral artery waveform

    D. None of the above

    E. A renal artery waveform

353. A popliteal to dorsal pedal lesser saphenous reverse bypass graft has a peak systolic velocity of 28 cm/sec at the distal anastomosis. Which of the following is true?

    A. This velocity may be normal for this graft.

    B. The graft is failing because the velocity is less than 45 cm/sec.

    C. The graft is failing because the graft velocity has increased from 24 cm/sec measured in a previous study.

    D. The graft is failing because the graft velocity has decreased from 32 cm/sec measured in a previous study.

    E. We must know the diastolic velocity before interpreting this velocity information.

354. The two flow characteristics that define arterial stenosis anywhere in the body include focal acceleration of velocities and:

    A. Decreased diastolic flow

    B. Decreased resistance proximally

    C. Increased flow reversal

    D. Increased pulsatility distally

    E. Distal turbulence

355. Diastolic reversal of flow is most likely in:

    A. The renal arteries
    B. The internal carotid artery
    C. Extremity arteries at rest
    D. Extremity arteries immediately following exercise
    E. The vena cava

356. Doppler velocity waveforms from upper extremity vessels may vary slightly from lower extremity waveforms because:

    A. The upstroke is not as sharp.
    B. The peripheral resistance is usually lower in the upper extremity.
    C. The peripheral resistance is usually higher in the upper extremity.
    D. There is never a diastolic flow reversal component at rest.
    E. B and D.

357. A 28-year-old male complains of exercise-induced cramping of the right calf that occurs after walking six blocks and is relieved within 5 minutes of rest. Bounding pedal pulses are noted and resting ankle pressures are normal. The symptoms are reproduced with exercise. The ankle pressure remains normal on the left but drops to 40 mmHg on the right. These signs are consistent with:

    A. Occlusion of the superficial femoral artery
    B. Compartment syndrome
    C. Popliteal entrapment
    D. Coarctation of the aorta
    E. Deep venous thrombosis

358. Your segmental pressure readings disclose a 36 mmHg decrease in pressure from the low-thigh to the below-knee anterior tibial artery, and a 10 mmHg decrease from low-thigh to below-knee posterior tibial artery. These findings localize obstruction to the:

    A. Distal superficial femoral artery
    B. Popliteal artery
    C. Posterior tibial artery
    D. Anterior tibial artery
    E. Peroneal artery

359. Your segmental pressure readings indicate 126 mmHg at the high thigh, 144 at the low thigh, and 120 at the below-knee level. These findings might be the result of all EXCEPT:

    A. SFA obstruction
    B. Cuff artifact
    C. Poor cuff application
    D. Calcified arteries in a diabetic patient
    E. All are possible causes

360. All of the following devices, utilized in a standard fashion, can measure ankle pressures EXCEPT:

    A. Doppler ultrasound

B. B-mode ultrasound
C. Strain-gauge plethysmography
D. Photocell plethysmography
E. Air plethysmography

361. This CW Doppler waveform from a popliteal artery:

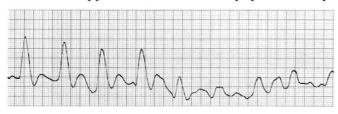

A. Is a normal arterial waveform
B. Is severely abnormal in character
C. Suggests interference from venous flow
D. Suggests femoral artery occlusion
E. Is monophasic

362. Protocols for cardiac treadmill testing and claudication treadmill testing differ, the major difference being:

A. A single, faster speed is used for cardiac testing.
B. The patient is closely monitored by technologists during cardiac testing.
C. Speed is varied during cardiac testing.
D. The cardiac risk is greater with claudication testing since few patients are monitored with ECG.
E. Elevation is varied during claudication testing.

363. A four-level pressure cuff technique is used to assess arterial disease in the legs. The high-thigh pressure is 140 mmHg, with an arm pressure of 160 mmHg. All of the following lesions can cause this EXCEPT:

A. Significant aortic stenosis
B. Common iliac or external iliac artery disease
C. Superficial femoral plus profunda artery occlusion
D. Common femoral artery disease
E. Isolated profunda femoral artery disease

364. While performing a treadmill test, the patient complains of pain in the left arm and jaw, but denies any other pain. The examiner should consider that this could possibly be:

A. Arm claudication
B. Angina
C. Unimportant symptoms
D. Subclavian steal
E. Carotid artery disease

365. During assessment of ankle pressures, all three vessels at the level of the ankle are used to measure pressures. The pressure in both the posterior tibial and peroneal artery is 40 mmHg and the dorsalis pedis pressure is 50mmHg. Which of the following is TRUE?

A. The posterior tibial artery pressure should be used to calculate the ankle/brachial index.
B. The dorsalis pedis artery pressure should be used to calculate the ankle/brachial index.
C. The peroneal artery pressure should be used to calculate the ankle/brachial index.
D. There is disease in the tibioperoneal trunk.
E. There is disease in or above the popliteal artery.

366. Your segmental pressure readings indicate the following:

Rt. brachial: 144 mmHg	Lt. Brachial: 140
Rt. high thigh: 110	Lt. high thigh: 164

These findings could result from all EXCEPT:

A. Aortoiliac obstruction
B. Right common iliac obstruction
C. Right external iliac obstruction
D. Right common femoral obstruction
E. Right proximal superficial femoral obstruction

367. Normal diameter for the abdominal aorta is:

A. Less than 1 cm
B. 2–3 cm
C. 3–5 cm
D. 5–7 cm
E. Approximately 10 cm

368. A patient complains of rest pain. On physical examination, elevation pallor and dependent rubor are present. There are no palpable pulses in the leg. A pressure of 120 mmHg is measured in the ankle. This pressure:

A. Is consistent with the patient presentation
B. Is lower than expected
C. Is higher than expected
D. Suggests the physical examination is erroneous
E. Obviates the need for arteriography

369. A patient with a history of rest pain, 100-foot calf and thigh claudication, and an ulcer on the great toe of the left foot has a left ankle pressure of >300 mmHg. This result is:

A. Diagnostic of a diabetic foot
B. Erroneous due to probable arterial calcification
C. Consistent with small vessel disease
D. Demonstrable of severe hypertension
E. Elevated due to a cuff that is too narrow

370. A patient with mild claudication-like symptoms has an ankle/brachial index for the affected leg of 1.02. This finding:

A. Indicates the disease is limited to the tibial arteries
B. Rules out the presence of any arterial disease

C. Is an incomplete evaluation of this patient

D. Demonstrates calcific arteries

E. Implicates neurogenic claudication as the cause of symptoms

371. After walking for 5 minutes on the treadmill, a patient experiences decreases in ankle pressure of 40% on the right and 15% on the left. These findings:

A. Suggest bilateral femoral artery occlusions

B. Suggest right femoral artery occlusion

C. Are within normal limits

D. Are typical for patients with claudication

E. Are not diagnostically useful

The following information applies to questions 372 and 373:

Right arm 180/100 mmHg
Left arm 120/60 mmHg
Right PTA 100 mmHg
Left PTA 90 mmHg

PTA = posterior tibial artery

---

372. The left ankle/brachial index is:

A. 0.50 (90/180)

B. 0.75 (90/120)

C. 0.90 (90/100)

D. 1.11 (100/90)

E. 1.50 (90/60)

373. In consideration of the aforementioned pressure findings, which of the following statements is NOT true?

A. The patient has right lower extremity arterial disease.

B. The patient has left lower extremity arterial disease.

C. The patient has left subclavian artery disease.

D. The patient has renovascular hypertension.

E. Arteriography would be recommended if bypass surgery is contemplated.

374. A male patient walks on the treadmill for an evaluation of leg symptoms. During the walk he reports that both calves and thighs start hurting at 10 seconds, the right worse than the left. He continues to walk for 5 minutes, after which he is stopped by the technologist. The symptoms do not resolve, but do not get worse during exercise. The following pressures are obtained:

Before exercise:
Arm 130   Right ankle 130   Left ankle 120

After exercise:
Arm 160   Right ankle 100   Left ankle 110

True statement(s) regarding this test is (are):

A. There is arterial disease in both legs.
B. The symptoms are probably not due to vascular disease.
C. The right leg is symptomatically worse.
D. There is evidence of aortoiliac artery disease.
E. A and B.
F. A and D.
G. A, B, and C.

375. A patient walks on the treadmill until forced to stop at 3 minutes due to left calf and thigh pain. The right leg was asymptomatic throughout the course of the testing. The following results were obtained:

Pre-exercise:
Right arm 150   Right PTA 120   Left PTA 120

Postexercise:
Right arm 150   Right PTA 75   Left PTA 50

PTA = posterior tibial artery

Which of the following statements is TRUE regarding this information?

A. There is arterial disease in both legs.
B. The left leg has worse disease than the right.
C. The patient has aortoiliac arterial disease.
D. Retesting the patient in 30 minutes should result in a shorter walking time.
E. The arm pressure normally increases after treadmill testing, raising questions of the validity of these results.
F. A and B.
G. C and D.
H. C and E.
I. This question has too many answers.

376. The correct setting for arterial volume recording is:

A. AC-coupled output
B. DC-coupled output
C. 3.5 Hz filter setting
D. "Mean" filter setting
E. Forward/reverse

377. Doppler waveform abnormalities in the lower extremity arterial circulation distal to a hemodynamically significant stenosis include:

A. Increased peak-to-peak amplitude
B. The presence of a dicrotic notch on the downslope
C. An absent flow reversal component, blunting of the peak velocity, and prolonged upslope and downslope
D. Absent Doppler signal
E. A triphasic waveform

378. Parameters usually assessed in exercise testing include all EXCEPT:

    A. Changes in thigh-to-ankle index
    B. Time required for recovery to pre-stress pressure level
    C. Patient complaint of leg pain during exercise
    D. Length of time of exercise
    E. Magnitude of pressure drop

379. Reasons to perform reactive hyperemia instead of treadmill testing include all EXCEPT:

    A. Patient's inability to tolerate application of pressure cuffs
    B. Patient's inability to stand or walk
    C. Patient's poor cardiac status
    D. Patient has pulmonary problems
    E. Patient has very severe disease in one leg, making exercise assessment of the other leg difficult

380. A normal arterial volume waveform may have all EXCEPT:

    A. Swift upstroke
    B. Sharp peak
    C. Rapid downslope bowed toward baseline
    D. Dicrotic notch
    E. Reverse-flow component

381. The most widely used interpretive technique for analog Doppler waveforms is:

    A. A quantitative approach evaluating the diagnostic features of the waveform
    B. A qualitative approach or pattern recognition
    C. Purely subjective (neither qualitative or quantitative information can be derived from the waveform)
    D. Spectral analysis of the velocity profiles within a waveform
    E. B-mode ultrasound evaluation

382. Normal Doppler waveform morphology for a peripheral artery includes:

    A. Phasicity with respiration
    B. Augmentation with distal compression maneuvers
    C. A sharp upslope and downslope and a prominent reverse flow component
    D. A delayed systolic peak with a downslope bowed away from the baseline
    E. A rounded, extended acceleration with no diastolic wave

383. A normal response of ankle pressure to exercise testing (such as treadmill) is:

    A. No change

B. A dramatic increase, 50% or more

C. A dramatic decrease, at least 50% in normals

D. A gradual decrease of 50% over five to ten minutes

E. A gradual increase of 50% over five to ten minutes

384. The amplitude of arterial volume recording waveforms:

A. Is identical at all four levels

B. Is highest distally, where hydrostatic pressure is highest

C. Is only marginally meaningful diagnostically

D. Is normally approximately one-third the width of the waveform

E. Should equal the reverse component

385. Possible error(s) that can occur when recording a femoral arterial waveform using continuous-wave Doppler include:

A. Insonating an artery other than the intended one

B. Recording two vessels simultaneously

C. Using an improper probe frequency

D. B and C only

E. All of the above

386. The Doppler beam may be attenuated if:

A. The sound beam must pass through scar tissue, a hematoma, or excessive fat

B. The vessel has calcific plaque on the anterior wall

C. Output settings from the Doppler to the recording device are not amplified

D. All the above

E. A and B only

387. With severe lower extremity arterial occlusive disease, the Doppler waveforms distally:

A. Will eventually return to a relatively normal waveform pattern once the disease process has stabilized

B. Will demonstrate flow reversal in the diastolic component

C. Cannot be distinguished from venous waveforms

D. Will appear markedly dampened, possibly making interpretation difficult for distal segments

E. Are almost always absent at the ankle level

388. Transcutaneous partial pressure of oxygen ($TcPO_2$) studies can be useful for all EXCEPT:

A. Determination of arterial level of obstruction

B. Determination of amputation level

C. Assessment of skin-graft viability

D. Assessment of foot perfusion

E. Assessment of healing of stump

389. The usual cuff pressure used in arterial volume recording is:

A. 65 mmHg

B. 10 mmHg

    C. Suprasystolic

    D. 100 mmHg

    E. Dependent on patient size

390. This digital photoplethysmographic waveform might suggest:

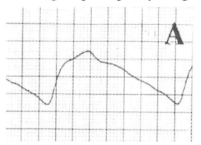

    A. Primary Raynaud's disease

    B. Secondary Raynaud's disease

    C. Venous valvular incompetence

    D. Nerve compression

    E. This is a normal digital PPG waveform

391. Distal to an aortoiliac occlusion, the common femoral artery signal is typically:

    A. Multiphasic

    B. Biphasic

    C. Low-pitched and monophasic

    D. Impossible to distinguish from a pulsatile venous signal

    E. High-pitched

392. Diastolic flow reversal:

    A. Is always present in all abnormal limbs

    B. Is always present in vasodilated limbs

    C. May be absent in vasodilated limbs

    D. Is absent in vasoconstricted limbs

    E. None of the above

393. The most important reason Doppler evaluations should be performed with the patient in a basal state and warm temperature is:

    A. The exam will be easier to perform.

    B. The results are influenced by the patient's peripheral resistance.

    C. The results can be expected to vary from day to day.

    D. The results are influenced by the pressure differential found in each vessel.

    E. Metabolic activity is increased, making results more reliable.

394. Audible Doppler venous signals typically are low-frequency and vary with respiration, whereas normal arterial signals in the legs and arms are:

    A. Low-frequency yet pulsatile

    B. Multiphasic and vary with respiration

    C. Relatively high-frequency with pulsatile components

    D. Relatively high-frequency and nonpulsatile

E. Multiphasic and phasic with respiration

395. If one is listening with a continuous-wave Doppler directly over a stenotic lesion, the signal will:

A. Be comprised of low-frequency flow disturbances
B. Have a distinct "thumping" sound
C. Be relatively unchanged from the rest of the vessel
D. Have a high-frequency sound
E. Be inaudible

396. Little or no increase of blood flow velocity in response to postocclusive reactive hyperemia (PORH), using an inflated thigh cuff, would most likely indicate:

A. An adequate, well-developed collateral bed
B. Significant obstructive disease
C. Small vessel disease in the foot
D. A normal arterial segment
E. Venous reconstitution

397. A normal postocclusive reactive hyperemia velocity response is:

A. A >100% increase in mean velocity
B. Approximately 50% increase in mean velocity
C. Any increase in mean velocity
D. An 80% decrease in mean velocity
E. No increase in mean velocity

398. Monophasic posterior tibial artery waveforms, despite normal ankle/arm indices in the asymptomatic patient, indicate that:

A. The low pass filter may be set too low.
B. The low pass filter may be set too high.
C. The Doppler gain may be set too high.
D. The angle of insonation may be too low.
E. The angle of insonation may be too high.

399. In a patient who wakes up at night with pain in the foot and has to drop the foot by the side of the bed, the ankle/arm systolic pressure ratio will most likely be:

A. Less than 0.50
B. Between 0.50 and 0.80
C. Between 0.80 and 1.00
D. Greater than 1.00
E. Not measurable

400. In the presence of tibial arterial calcification in the diabetic patient, the ankle/arm index:

A. Is reliable unless immeasurable because of arterial incompressibility
B. Cannot be in the normal range
C. May be in the normal range or abnormally decreased, yet falsely elevated
D. Is always nondiagnostic

E. May be in the abnormal range yet falsely reduced

401. You are performing CW Doppler on a patient's lower extremity arteries. You obtain a signal at the proximal dorsalis pedis level. When you move proximally, the signal becomes higher in pitch. This could be the result of all EXCEPT:

A. You have moved over a stenotic area.
B. You have stood the probe up, increasing the angle of incidence.
C. You have leaned the probe back, decreasing the angle of incidence.
D. You have moved over a segment of the artery which is going deeper.
E. You are pushing too hard on the probe, artificially narrowing the artery under it.

402. While monitoring of femorodistal bypass graft using duplex ultrasonography, the graft may be at risk of failure if:

A. The graft velocity is more than 45 cm/sec.
B. The graft velocity is 130 cm/sec.
C. The graft velocity has been around 30 cm/sec for over three years since its implantation.
D. The graft velocity has dropped from 70 cm/sec, as measured 6 months earlier, to 30 cm/sec.
E. The ankle blood pressure stays the same.

403. Toe pressures:

A. Are falsely elevated as frequently as tibial ankle pressures
B. Are falsely elevated less frequently than tibial ankle pressures
C. Are falsely elevated more frequently than tibial ankle pressures
D. Are falsely decreased due to arterial incompressibility
E. Cannot be measured in the presence of tibial artery incompressibility

404. Systolic thigh pressures are 180 mmHg in both lower extremities; the systolic arm pressure is 170 mmHg on the right and 160 mmHg on the left. The patient complains of buttock claudication.

A. The patient does not have significant aortoiliac occlusive disease because the thigh pressures are normal.
B. The patient does not have unilateral iliac occlusive disease because the thigh pressures are normal and equal.
C. The patient has bilateral superficial femoral artery occlusion.
D. Thigh pressures are not used to determine the presence of iliac occlusive disease.
E. The patient may have aortoiliac occlusive disease.

405. Systolic thigh pressures could be accurately measured with standard (12 cm wide) arm cuffs:

A. In all patients
B. In patients with large thighs
C. In patients with similar thigh and arm diameters
D. In all patients without arterial incompressibility
E. In no patients

406. To minimize error during the measurement of the systolic pressures using a manometer having 2 mmHg marks, the deflation rate should be:

    A. Approximately 5 mmHg per second
    B. Less than 1 mmHg per second
    C. Varies with the severity of the disease
    D. Approximately 2 mmHg per heart beat
    E. Depends on the size of the cuff

407. A PTFE graft can be identified during ultrasonographic imaging by:

    A. A zigzag appearance of the graft walls
    B. A double-line appearance of the graft walls
    C. A single-line appearance of the graft walls
    D. A distinct color pattern
    E. The graft cannot be identified ultrasonographically

408. A patient has a 50% diameter stenosis in a lower extremity vein graft. The systolic velocity at the stenosis:

    A. Will be 50% higher than the prestenotic velocity
    B. Is greater than 150 cm/sec, less than 240 cm/sec
    C. Is less than 45 cm/sec
    D. Is the same as the velocities measured distally in the graft
    E. Will be 100% greater than the prestenotic velocity followed by a drop in velocity

409. The velocities measured in a reversed saphenous vein bypass graft are usually:

    A. Higher proximally and lower distally
    B. Lower proximally and higher distally
    C. The same throughout the graft
    D. Greater than 100 cm/sec throughout the graft
    E. Unreliable due to vein-wall differences relative to a native artery

410. The volume flow rate in a reversed saphenous vein bypass graft should be:

    A. Higher proximally and lower distally
    B. Lower proximally and higher distally
    C. The same throughout the graft
    D. Variable throughout the graft
    E. Inversely proportional to the diameter of the graft

411. In the presence of arterial obstructive disease and distal ischemia:

    A. Vasoconstriction increases, and distal resistance increases.
    B. Vasoconstriction increases, and distal resistance decreases.
    C. Vasodilatation decreases, and distal resistance decreases.
    D. Vasodilatation increases, and distal resistance decreases.
    E. Vasodilatation decreases, and distal resistance may either increase or remain the same.

412. A damped Doppler velocity waveform of the subclavian artery isolates a significant lesion:

   A. At or distal to the brachial artery

   B. Proximal to the point of insonation

   C. Near the origin of the subclavian artery

   D. To the vertebral artery

   E. To the innominate artery

413. Normal values in $TcPO_2$ assessment are:

   A. Not yet established

   B. 60–80 mmHg

   C. Approximately 760 mmHg (atmospheric pressure)

   D. 10–20 mmHg

   E. 0 mmHg, changing to 10–20 mmHg with O_2 challenge

414. Evaluation of an abdominal aortic aneurysm is facilitated if the study is done:

   A. After lunch but before dinner

   B. After breakfast but before lunch

   C. Before breakfast

   D. After dinner

   E. This study does not depend on patient preparation.

415. Which set of waveforms is most likely to be obtained with a continuous-wave Doppler when there is a long superficial femoral artery occlusion?

   A. Triphasic waveforms from the common femoral to the tibial arteries

   B. Triphasic waveforms at the common femoral and proximal superficial femoral arteries with monophasic waveforms in the popliteal and tibial arteries

   C. Monophasic waveforms throughout

   D. Monophasic waveforms at the popliteal artery and triphasic waveforms at the tibial arteries

   E. Triphasic waveforms at the femoropopliteal arteries and monophasic waveforms at the tibial arteries

416. In the calculation of ankle/brachial systolic pressure ratios, the following arm pressure is commonly selected as the denominator:

   A. The higher of the right or left arm pressures

   B. The lower of the right or left arm pressures

   C. The right arm pressure

   D. The left arm pressure

   E. Random selection of the right or left arm pressure

417. Match the symptoms with the likely ankle/arm index:

   1. Claudication   a. ABI > 1.30

   2. Rest pain   b. ABI between 1.00 and 1.30

                    c. ABI between 0.5 and 0.80

                    d. ABI < 0.50

A. 1-b and 2-c
B. 1-b and 2-d
C. 1-c and 2-d
D. 1-c and 2-a
E. 1-a and 2-d

418. A normal ankle-pressure response to reactive hyperemia is:

A. A gradual decrease of approximately 50%
B. A quick, transient drop of greater than 50%
C. A transient decrease of approximately 20%
D. A transient increase of approximately 50%
E. A gradual increase of approximately 50%

419. Which technique is LEAST likely to be used to record digital pulses or changes in arterial volume?

A. Air plethysmography
B. Duplex ultrasonography
C. Pneumatic technique
D. Strain gauge
E. Photoplethysmography

420. Pulse volume recordings demonstrate a lack of dicrotic notch in the recordings at the thigh, decreased pulses at the upper calf, and flat tracings at the ankle. The most likely interpretation of this study is:

A. Mild iliofemoral, superficial femoral, and tibial artery occlusive disease
B. Mild iliofemoral, superficial femoral, and severe tibial artery occlusive disease
C. Severe iliofemoral, superficial femoral, and tibial artery occlusive disease
D. Mild iliofemoral stenosis, severe superficial femoral stenosis or occlusion, and severe infrapopliteal occlusive disease
E. Aortic occlusion

421. In a study of the upper extremities, pulse volume recordings show lack of dicrotic notch at all levels of a patient with warm hands and fingers bilaterally. The patient:

A. Has bilateral subclavian artery stenoses
B. Has a lacunar stroke
C. Is vasodilated
D. Has had a sympathectomy in the past
E. Is vasoconstricted

422. A clenched fist will change the following parameter in the brachial artery Doppler waveform:

A. Increase the pulsatility index
B. Decrease the pulsatility index
C. Increase diastolic flow
D. Decrease systolic flow
E. Increase the average velocity

423. Which statement probably does NOT describe aspects of Raynaud's disease?

    A. Normal digital pressures when the hand is immersed in cold water.
    B. Decreased pressures when the hand is immersed in cold water.
    C. Normal wrist pressures when the hand is immersed in cold water.
    D. Sequential white, blue, then eventually red color changes in fingers when the hand is immersed in cold water.
    E. Sequential white, blue, then eventually red color changes in toes when the foot is immersed in cold water.

424. A 12-year-old is noted by the pediatrician to have decreased femoral artery pulses and is referred to the laboratory for evaluation. Bilateral arm blood pressures are 210/100, and femoral artery pulses bilaterally are indeed diminished, as are the ankle pressures. Femoral artery Doppler waveforms are abnormal. The diagnosis that should be entertained in this child is:

    A. Aortoiliac occlusive disease
    B. Coarctation of the aorta
    C. Compartment syndrome
    D. Patent ductus arteriosus
    E. Renal artery stenosis

425. Which statement is correct regarding digital subtraction arteriography (DSA)?

    A. The contrast is injected into the veins, not in the arteries.
    B. DSA has a larger field of view than standard angiography.
    C. DSA automatically selects for subtraction two or three frames obtained during injection of contrast solution.
    D. A mask, often without contrast, is selected to be subtracted from the frames obtained during injection of the contrast solution.
    E. In modern instruments, the bony landmarks are lost and not recoverable during subtraction.

426. Which of the following is a significant problem with digital subtraction angiography?

    A. Longer than normal procedure time
    B. Increase in contrast dosage
    C. Single view filming technique
    D. Patient cooperation
    E. Inability to provide sequential images

427. Which of the following is NOT correct regarding peripheral arterial angiography?

    A. It is frequently used prior to elective operation for peripheral arterial occlusive disease.
    B. There are problems with vessel overlap using angiography.
    C. Arteriography is used for routine postoperative follow-up.
    D. Contrast reactions are less of a problem than in years past.
    E. Digital subtraction angiography may be performed with intravenous or intraarterial injections.

428. The usual site of puncture for percutaneous lower extremity (or any) angiography is:

    A. Axillary artery
    B. Common femoral artery
    C. Posterior tibial artery
    D. Internal jugular vein
    E. Brachial artery

429. The common radiologic terms "inflow, outflow, runoff" refer respectively to:

    A. Arterial side, capillaries, and venous side
    B. Right heart, pulmonary bed, and systemic circulation
    C. Arterial side, venous side, and perforating veins
    D. Aortoiliac, femoropopliteal, and trifurcation arteries
    E. Upper extremity, lower extremity, and torso arteries

430. Arteriography would be contraindicated or approached very cautiously in a patient with:

    A. Diabetes mellitus
    B. Renal failure
    C. Cancer
    D. Peripheral vascular disease
    E. Mad cow disease

431. The condition which typically shows up on angiography as a "string of beads" is:

    A. Diabetes mellitus
    B. Raynaud's syndrome
    C. Takayasu's arteritis
    D. Polyarteritis nodosa
    E. Fibromuscular dysplasia

432. Computed tomography is useful in the lower extremities primarily for detection of:

    A. Arterial occlusion
    B. Venous thrombosis
    C. Femoral or popliteal aneurysm
    D. Arteriovenous malformation
    E. Esophageal varices

433. Regarding the use of magnetic resonance arteriography (MRA) for evaluation of lower extremity arteries, which is FALSE?

    A. MRA cannot achieve the accuracy of conventional angiography.
    B. MRA does not have the potential side effects that conventional angiography entails.
    C. MRA is more sensitive than conventional angiography in identifying patent runoff arteries.
    D. MRA is more cost-effective than conventional angiography.
    E. MRA can be used alone before bypass surgery (without conventional angiography).

434. Compared to patency rates in the iliac arteries, patency rates for angioplasty of the infrainguinal arteries are:

A. Better
B. Worse
C. Approximately equal
D. Angioplasty is not performed on infrainguinal arteries
E. Angioplasty is not performed on iliac or infrainguinal arteries

435. The "kissing stent" angioplasty/stent technique is useful for:

A. Renal arteries
B. The adductor canal region
C. Total occlusions
D. Infrarenal arteries only
E. Bifurcations

436. The type of revascularization surgery that requires the use of a valvulatome is:

A. In situ saphenous graft
B. Reversed saphenous graft
C. End-to-side synthetic graft
D. Side-to-side synthetic graft
E. Graft vein taken from upper extremity

437. The upper extremity vein most commonly used for an arterial bypass in the leg is the:

A. Cephalic vein
B. Basilic vein
C. Brachial vein
D. Axillary vein
E. Radial vein

438. Which superficial vein is NOT commonly used as a bypass graft?

A. The great saphenous vein
B. The small saphenous vein
C. The basilic vein
D. The cephalic vein
E. The femoral vein

439. A patient has a 7 cm abdominal aortic aneurysm. The patient elects not to have an operation, despite the surgeon's recommendation. Which of the following statements is FALSE?

A. The mortality of rupture, even with prompt care, is at least 50%.
B. The risk of death from cardiac disease is greater than the risk of death from rupture of the aneurysm.
C. There is little risk for distal embolization.
D. There is little risk for aortic occlusion.
E. The surgeon's recommendation is sound based on the natural history of AAA.

440. A 64-year-old male complains of half-block left thigh and calf claudication without symptoms on the right. Physical examination reveals that the left femoral pulse is absent;

pulses on the right are normal, without bruit. Treadmill testing results are abnormal on the left, normal on the right. Duplex reveals an occluded iliac artery on the left. This patient may be an ideal candidate for:

A. Femorofemoral bypass
B. Axillofemoral bypass
C. Balloon angioplasty
D. Femoropopliteal bypass
E. Lumbar sympathectomy

441. The five-year risk for rupture of abdominal aortic aneurysms of 4 cm is approximately:

A. >50%
B. 40%
C. 30%
D. 20%
E. <10%

442. Regarding lumbar sympathectomy, all are true EXCEPT:

A. Potentially useful in patients with Raynaud's disease
B. Potentially useful in patients with ischemic rest pain
C. Unlikely to be useful in patients with ischemic ulceration
D. Potentially useful in claudicating patients
E. Increases vasodilatation and blood flow primarily in cutaneous vascular beds

443. The most effective lytic treatment for acute arterial thrombosis is:

A. tPA
B. Heparin
C. Sodium warfarin
D. Vasopressors
E. Inotropic agents

444. Your measurement of a patient's abdominal aorta gives a diameter of 6.5 cm. The probable management of this patient would involve:

A. Elective repair
B. Percutaneous angioplasty
C. Follow-up scan in one year
D. Endarterectomy
E. No course of action; this finding is within normal limits

PART V

Abdominal & Visceral Vascular Disease

Mechanisms of Abdominal and Visceral Vascular Disease

Signs and Symptoms of Abdominal and Visceral Vascular Disease

Testing and Treatment of Abdominal and Visceral Vascular Disease

MECHANISMS OF ABDOMINAL AND VISCERAL VASCULAR DISEASE

Risk factors

Renovascular hypertension

Mesenteric ischemia

Portal hypertension

445. You are performing a Doppler exam on a patient with suspected renovascular hypertension. Which diagnostic parameter is the best indicator of renovascular disease?

   A. Pulsatility index

   B. A/B ratio

   C. Renal/aortic ratio

   D. Systolic/diastolic ratio

   E. None of the above

446. The abdominal vessel that is most commonly compromised by compression of the median arcuate ligament of the diaphragm is the:

   A. Inferior vena cava

   B. Left gastric artery

   C. Superior mesenteric artery

   D. Celiac artery

   E. None of the above

447. What is the most common location of atherosclerotic disease of the renal artery?

   A. Proximal

   B. Mid

   C. Distal

   D. Intrarenal

   E. The disease strikes all of these sites with about the same frequency.

448. Which of the following is NOT a common feature of renal allograft rejection?

A. Increased allograft size
B. Increased cortical echogenicity
C. Decreased flow resistance in parenchymal arteries
D. Increased prominence of the renal pyramids
E. All are common features of rejection.

449. In a patient with portal hypertension, the most likely result of increased portal venous pressure would be:

A. Cavernous transformation
B. Aortic dissection
C. Hepatic artery aneurysm
D. Enlarged coronary vein
E. Each of these results is equally likely.

450. A spontaneous splenorenal shunt—an abnormal connection between the splenic vein and the left renal vein—is associated with:

A. Renovascular hypertension
B. Portal hypertension
C. Renal failure
D. Renal cell carcinoma
E. Acute IVC thrombosis

451. The Budd-Chiari syndrome is a cause of portal hypertension resulting from:

A. Hepatic artery stenosis
B. Inferior mesenteric vein thrombus
C. Superior vena cava thrombus
D. Hepatic vein obstruction
E. A liver tumor

452. In the United States the most common cause of portal hypertension is:

A. Hepatic carcinoma
B. Cirrhosis
C. Hypertension
D. Schistosomiasis
E. Hyperlipidemia

453. To evaluate blood flow within the splanchnic arteries, you should examine the following vessels:

A. Celiac artery, superior mesenteric artery, inferior mesenteric artery
B. Main portal vein, right portal vein, left portal vein
C. Right and left renal arteries and veins
D. Right and left common iliac and external iliac arteries
E. All of the above

SIGNS & SYMPTOMS OF ABDOMINAL AND VISCERAL VASCULAR DISEASE

454. The patient with advanced chronic mesenteric ischemia is most likely to be:

    A. Obese
    B. Malnourished
    C. In atrial fibrillation
    D. Hyperactive
    E. Free of discernable symptoms

455. Patients with significant mesenteric artery obstructive disease generally have symptoms of:

    A. Preprandial pain, relieved by eating.
    B. Preprandial bloating, relieved by eating.
    C. Postprandial pain.
    D. Postprandial syncope.
    E. Postprandial hypertensive state.

456. Patients being evaluated for portal hypertension may have liver-dysfunction symptoms including all of the following EXCEPT:

    A. Jaundice
    B. Clotting abnormalities
    C. Malnutrition
    D. Ascites
    E. Claudication

457. A common manifestation of portal hypertension is:

    A. Claudication
    B. Vasculogenic impotence
    C. Bleeding esophageal varices
    D. Homonymous hemianopia
    E. Clubbing of digits

458. You are examining a patient who presents with weight loss, postprandial pain, and an abdominal bruit. Obstruction of which vessel is most likely to be at least partly responsible for these symptoms?

    A. Portal vein
    B. Renal arteries
    C. Superior mesenteric artery
    D. Splenic vein
    E. None of the above

459. The patient you are scanning has an enlarged coronary vein with retrograde flow. These findings are a sign of:

    A. Renal parenchymal disease
    B. Thrombosis of the inferior vena cava
    C. Iliac vein thrombus
    D. Portal hypertension
    E. Thrombosis of the renal vein

TESTING & TREATMENT OF ABDOMINAL AND VISCERAL VASCULAR DISEASE

Duplex imaging

Angiography

Treatment

460. Noninvasive diagnosis of renal artery stenosis:

    A. Can be made by B-mode images of atherosclerotic plaque
    B. Cannot be made since the renal arteries are too deep for ultrasound penetration
    C. Requires a duplex system with spectral signal analysis
    D. Can be accomplished with a non-duplex Doppler system
    E. Requires spiral CT technology

461. The abdominal artery that normally demonstrates higher diastolic flow postprandially is:

    A. Celiac axis
    B. Common hepatic
    C. Splenic
    D. Renal
    E. Superior mesenteric

462. Normal arterial waveforms in the renal hilum:

    A. Are phasic with respiration
    B. Are high-resistance in character (little diastolic flow)
    C. Are low-resistance in character (much diastolic flow)
    D. Cannot be obtained with duplex instrumentation
    E. Cycle with right-atrial activity

463. Proximal renal artery stenosis greater than 60% is diagnosed when:

    A. Systolic renal velocities are greater than 100 cm/sec
    B. Systolic renal velocities are less than 45 cm/sec
    C. Systolic renal/aortic velocity ratio is less than 3.5
    D. Systolic renal/aortic velocity ratio is greater than 3.5
    E. Stenoses are measured in real-time image, not extrapolated from velocities

464. In a patient with intestinal ischemia, the cause might be revealed by a duplex scan finding of stenoses in the following arteries:

    A. Right and left renal arteries
    B. Superior and inferior mesenteric artery
    C. The splenic and superior mesenteric artery
    D. Aorta and superior mesenteric artery
    E. Aorta and inferior mesenteric artery

465. A validated laboratory index for detection of significant renal artery stenosis is:

    A. Renal stenosis/aorta peak systolic velocity ratio greater than 1.8
    B. Renal stenosis/contralateral renal peak systolic velocity ratio greater than 3.5
    C. Renal stenosis peak systolic frequencies greater than 4.5 MHz
    D. Renal stenosis peak systolic velocity greater than 127 cm/sec
    E. Renal stenosis/aorta peak systolic velocity ratio greater than 3.5

466. With inspiration, a Doppler signal from the subclavian vein will usually:

    A. Augment
    B. Diminish
    C. Change direction
    D. Not respond
    E. Become biphasic

467. Pulsatile venous Doppler from the portal vein may suggest:

    A. Cardiac dysrhythmia
    B. Portal hypertension
    C. Respiratory variations
    D. Hepatic artery obstruction
    E. Normal flow

468. In duplex assessment of the portal vein, flow:

    A. Normally is phasic with respiration
    B. Normally is continuous with respiration
    C. Is minimally altered during portal hypertension
    D. Is minimally diverted from the liver with portocaval shunt
    E. Is minimally modulated by abdominal pressure

469. A normal spectral waveform from the hepatic veins is:

    A. Continuous
    B. Unidirectional
    C. Bidirectional
    D. Triphasic
    E. A and B

470. Demonstration of vein-wall coaptation of the subclavian vein is best performed with:

   A. Probe compression (as in the lower extremities)
   B. Firm arm compression
   C. The patient taking a quick, deep breath
   D. The Valsalva maneuver
   E. The subclavian vein cannot be assessed for vein-wall coaptation.

471. A Doppler signal from the subclavian vein is expected normally to be:

   A. Triphasic
   B. Pulsatile
   C. Absent in older patients
   D. Nonspontaneous except in warm patients
   E. Retrograde

472. Normal flow in the hepatic vein is:

   A. Hepatopetal
   B. Retrograde
   C. Triphasic
   D. Bidirectional
   E. Not detectable with duplex

473. Which vessel would be imaged in a patient referred to rule out Budd-Chiari syndrome?

   A. Innominate vein
   B. Internal jugular vein
   C. Hepatic vein
   D. Common femoral vein
   E. Circumflex vein

474. Which of the following is a normal finding in a patient who has a transjugular intrahepatic portosystemic shunt (TIPS)?

   A. Hepatofugal flow in the main portal vein
   B. Hepatopetal flow in the main portal vein
   C. Hepatofugal flow in the splenic vein
   D. Absence of flow in the portal vein
   E. A, B, and C

475. In the preceding question, which disorder would necessitate the TIPS?

   A. Cirrhosis
   B. Multiple episodes of pulmonary embolus
   C. Splenomegaly
   D. Diabetes
   E. Myocardial infarction

PART VI

Miscellaneous Conditions & Tests

Preoperative Vein Mapping

Pseudoaneurysms, Arteriovenous Fistulae

Dialysis Access

Organ Transplants

Impotence Testing

Preoperative Arterial Mapping

Temporal Arteritis

Thoracic Outlet Syndrome

Trauma

476. Points of technique to be observed during ultrasound-guided compression of pseudoaneurysm include all EXCEPT:

A. Use color flow to confirm that flow remains biphasic within the pseudoaneurysm.
B. Monitor ankle pressure.
C. Use color flow to monitor flow in the common femoral artery.
D. Release pressure for a short time at 10 to 15 minute intervals.
E. Use color flow to confirm that flow is obliterated in the pseudoaneurysm.

477. The incidence of pseudoaneurysms is:

A. Increasing
B. Decreasing
C. Staying the same
D. Stabilizing
E. Not associated with iatrogenic causes

478. Which of the following is a TRUE statement regarding impotence?

A. Few impotent males have vascular disease as the etiology.
B. Penile pressure can decrease after treadmill testing.
C. Occlusions of the common iliac artery cannot cause vascular impotence.
D. Vascular impotence is almost always surgically correctable.
E. Erection is impossible if vascular impotence is present.

479. A uniform forearm cephalic vein measuring 2 mm in diameter during ultrasonographic imaging is being considered for a popliteal tibial bypass:

A. The vein could not be used because its diameter is less than 4 mm.

B. The vein could not be used because its diameter in the arm is 2 mm.

C. A uniform cephalic vein could not be used as a popliteal tibial bypass.

D. The vein could be used because the graft diameter must be 4 mm.

E. The vein might be used because the graft diameter is 2 mm and might expand under pressure.

480. While performing an abdominal ultrasound on a kidney transplant, you find that the renal artery and vein are patent, but the arteries of the transplanted kidney do not have diastolic flow. Which statement is true?

A. Lack of systolic flow is normal for the kidney.

B. Lack of diastolic flow is normal for the transplanted kidney.

C. Lack of diastolic flow is abnormal for the transplanted kidney.

D. Lack of diastolic flow is to be expected in the immediate post-transplantation period.

E. Diastolic flow does not provide useful information in the study of the kidneys.

481. A normal penile/brachial systolic pressure ratio is:

A. > 3.5:1

B. > 0.45

C. > 1.3

D. > 0.5

E. > 0.75

482. The proximal common femoral artery has high diastolic flow but the distal common femoral artery has a significantly increased reverse flow. The noninvasive study was performed after cardiac catheterization. The likely cause of these findings is:

A. Pseudoaneurysm that can be compressed with the probe

B. Pseudoaneurysm that is too large to be compressed by the probe

C. Arteriovenous fistula

D. Superficial femoral occlusion

E. Distal vasodilatation

483. A probe in the 7 to 10 MHz range is best used for:

A. Saphenous vein mapping prior to bypass surgery

B. Routine DVT studies in the lower extremity

C. Abdominal imaging

D. Cardiac echo

E. This is not a useful probe frequency for vascular studies.

484. An abnormal flow rate for a radial artery/cephalic vein dialysis fistula is:

A. 200 to 400 ml/min

B. 400 to 900 ml/min

C. 1000 to 1500 ml/min

D. Greater than 1500 ml/min

E. Less than 200 ml/min

485. The name for the type of graft described in the previous question is:

    A. Budd-Chiari
    B. Swan-Ganz
    C. McNeil-Lehrer
    D. PTFE
    E. Cimino-Brescia

486. The digital/brachial systolic pressure ratio in an extremity with a dialysis fistula usually is:

    A. Greater than 1.00
    B. About 0.80
    C. About 0.50
    D. Less than 0.50
    E. Should not be measured

487. A traumatic arteriovenous fistula produces:

    A. High diastolic arterial flow in the arteries distal to the fistula
    B. High, pulsatile venous flow in the veins distal to the fistula
    C. High, pulsatile venous flow in the veins proximal to the fistula
    D. Low systolic flow in the arteries proximal to the fistula
    E. Low, continuous flow in the veins proximal to the fistula

488. In the situation in the previous question, pressure in the artery distal to the fistula will be:

    A. Reduced
    B. Increased
    C. Variously increased or decreased depending on cardiac output
    D. Unchanged
    E. Immeasurable

489. A congenital arteriovenous fistula involves:

    A. A single arteriovenous pair
    B. Being easily occluded with microspheres
    C. Being easily ligated surgically
    D. A multitude of arteriovenous channels
    E. The lymphatic channels

490. In duplex assessment of dialysis fistulas (synthetic or native), common abnormalities include all EXCEPT:

    A. High flow rates exceeding 300 ml/min
    B. Stenosis at the venous anastomosis
    C. Aneurysm of the graft
    D. False aneurysm caused by needle puncture
    E. Spontaneous thrombosis

491. Anterior compartment syndrome is suspected in a trauma patient with closed fracture of the fibula. Clinically the calf is tense and tender to palpation, and there is decreased sensation in the foot. The dorsalis pedis pulse is present, with an audible triphasic Doppler signal.

The dorsalis pedis pressure is 140 mmHg, with an arm pressure of 130 mmHg. Why is this finding unreliable for ruling out a compartment syndrome?

A. Dorsalis pedis flow is not via the anterior tibial compartment, thus one would not expect the signal to be altered.

B. The posterior tibial or peroneal artery may supply collateral flow, such that the dorsalis pedis artery is unaffected.

C. Nerve and/or motor dysfunction due to compartment syndrome may occur without any alteration of arterial hemodynamics.

D. Compartment syndrome is not related to closed fractures.

E. The noninvasive arterial testing is inadequate. Venous testing would be necessary to make the diagnosis.

492. The disease/syndrome associated with compression of subclavian artery and brachial plexus by the cervical rib is:

A. Subclavian steal syndrome
B. Cervical spine disease
C. Thoracic outlet syndrome
D. Causalgia
E. Vertebral stenosis

493. Maneuvers used to assess the patient with possible thoracic outlet syndrome include all EXCEPT:

A. Hyperabduction of arms
B. Adson maneuver
C. Hobbs maneuver
D. Costoclavicular maneuver
E. Positioning to reproduce symptoms

494. The internal mammary artery is a branch of the:

A. Innominate artery
B. Subclavian artery
C. Vertebral artery
D. Axillary artery
E. Aorta

495. Temporal arteritis is commonly characterized by:

A. Dissection
B. Aneurysm
C. Intimal thickening
D. Tortuosity
E. Ectasia

496. In liver transplants, the native common hepatic artery is anastomosed to the donor hepatic artery:

A. In the posterior aspect of the right lobe of the liver
B. In the medial segment of the left lobe of the liver

C. Several centimeters proximal to the hepatic hilum
D. At the porta hepatis where the hepatic artery enters the liver
E. None of the above

497. While mapping the saphenous vein in a patient scheduled for coronary artery bypass operation, you discover that the saphenous veins are not adequate for harvesting. Which of the following veins would be best to evaluate as an alternate graft?

A. Cephalic vein
B. Deep femoral vein
C. Popliteal vein
D. Axillary vein
E. B, C, or D

498. Which of the following techniques would be most helpful in mapping the saphenous vein?

A. Decrease room temperature to dilate the small saphenous vein.
B. Place the patient in an upright position to improve visualization of the saphenous vein.
C. Place the patient in a prone position to improve access to the saphenous vein.
D. Use a high-frequency probe and light probe pressure to track the saphenous vein.
E. Use a lower-frequency probe and firm probe pressure to track the saphenous vein most effectively.

PART VII

Quality Assurance

Statistics

Patient Safety

499. The probability that a positive noninvasive test reveals actual disease (as diagnosed by the gold-standard test) is called:

   A. Accuracy
   B. Sensitivity
   C. Specificity
   D. Positive predictive value
   E. Negative predictive value

500. If we increase the peak systolic velocity value needed to call a carotid test positive for severe ICA stenosis:

   A. The positive predictive value will decrease, the negative predictive value will increase, and the accuracy may increase or decrease.
   B. The positive predictive value will increase, the negative predictive value will decrease, and the accuracy may increase or decrease.
   C. The positive predictive value and the accuracy will increase, and the negative predictive value will decrease.
   D. The negative predictive value and the accuracy will increase, and the positive predictive value will decrease.
   E. The positive and negative predictive values and the accuracy will remain the same.

501. Given the following information, overall accuracy can be:

Sensitivity = 91.3%
Specificity = 83.4%
Positive predictive value = 94.3%
Negative predictive value = 80.7%

   A. 78%
   B. 82%
   C. 85%
   D. 93%
   E. 96%

The following problem applies to questions 502–504:

Four hundred patients underwent noninvasive venous testing with subsequent venography. The noninvasive and venographic results were compared. Of the 300 normal venograms, 15 were abnormal by noninvasive testing. Of the 100 abnormal venograms, 90 were abnormal by noninvasive testing.

502. Overall accuracy is:

    A. 105/400
    B. 105/300
    C. 375/400
    D. 295/300
    E. 295/400

503. Sensitivity is:

    A. 15/300
    B. 15/400
    C. 105/400
    D. 375/400
    E. 90/100

504. Positive predictive value is:

    A. 90/105
    B. 90/400
    C. 100/400
    D. 375/400
    E. 390/400

505. The calculation that has as its denominator the total number of normal noninvasive tests is:

    A. Positive predictive value
    B. Sensitivity
    C. Overall accuracy
    D. Specificity
    E. Negative predictive value

506. For a correlation of carotid angiography and noninvasive carotid testing the specificity was calculated at 94.6% and the sensitivity was calculated at 90.3%. The overall accuracy can be:

    A. 24.3%
    B. 88.5%
    C. 92.3%

D. 94.6%

E. 95.1%

The following problem applies to questions 507–509:

A series of carotid duplex studies was correlated to carotid angiography to test a velocity threshold for accuracy in calling >60% vs. <60% stenosis of the internal carotid artery. Of the 56 ICAs called >60% by angiography, 53 were correctly identified by duplex. Of the 38 ICAs called <60% by angiography, 8 were called >60% by duplex.

---

507. The correct calculation for the positive predictive value is:

    A. 53/61

    B. 30/33

    C. 83/94

    D. 53/56

    E. 53/94

508. The correct calculation of specificity would be obtained by which of the following?

    A. 8/38

    B. 30/94

    C. 83/94

    D. 30/38

    E. 30/33

509. Which of the following statements about the aforementioned calculations is correct?

    A. The overall accuracy is less than either the positive or negative predictive values.

    B. The overall accuracy is greater than either the sensitivity or the specificity.

    C. The specificity is greater than the sensitivity.

    D. The specificity is greater than the positive predictive value.

    E. The negative predictive value is greater than the positive predictive value.

510. The customary format for the 2 x 2 table places the false positives in the:

    A. Upper left box

    B. Lower left box

    C. Upper right box

    D. Lower right box

    E. Center box

511. The 2 x 2 table below correlates arteriographically proven disease in the lower extremity arteries and a significant gradient in systolic pressure between segmental pressure cuffs.

Significant obstruction
by angiography

	Present	Absent
>20 mmHg	90	10
<20 mmHg	10	90

Pressure gradient between cuffs

All of the following are true EXCEPT:

A. Specificity and sensitivity are equal.
B. Positive and negative predictive values are equal.
C. Specificity and positive predictive value are equal.
D. Sensitivity and negative predictive value are equal.
E. Overall accuracy is calculated by the formula 90/100.

512. A correlation of a noninvasive test to its "gold standard" yields a positive predictive value of 86%. This means that:

A. Of all noninvasive tests performed, 86% correctly classified the disease.
B. Of all gold standard results that were abnormal, the noninvasive test correctly classified 86%.
C. Of all positive noninvasive tests, 86% correctly predicted that the gold standard would be abnormal.
D. Of all noninvasive tests performed, 86% were positive.
E. Of all positive noninvasive tests, 14 incorrectly predicted the gold standard would be abnormal.

513. A correlation of a noninvasive test to its gold standard yields a sensitivity of 93%. Which of the following statements regarding the specificity is correct?

A. It must be greater than the sensitivity.
B. It must be less than the sensitivity.
C. It must be equal to the sensitivity.
D. It must be within 10 to 15% of the sensitivity.
E. It must be a value from 0 to 100%.

514. The 2 x 2 table below shows data used to correlate ankle pressure measurement with healing in patients undergoing toe amputation.

	Not healed	Healed
<60 mmHg	15	3
>60 mmHg	5	27

ANKLE PRESSURE

The gold standard is healing of the amputation site. For the purposes of this study, a positive (abnormal) ankle pressure was < 60 mmHg. Which of the following statements is true?

A. The denominator for calculating sensitivity is 18.
B. The denominator for calculating specificity is 32.
C. The denominator for calculating overall accuracy is 42.
D. The denominator for calculating positive predictive value is 18.
E. The denominator for calculating negative predictive value is 30.

515. On the basis of the information in the preceding 2 x 2 table, the positive predictive value of the <60 mmHg threshold is calculated:

A. 15/20
B. 27/30
C. 27/32
D. 15/18
E. 42/50

After completing the study, the authors decided to review their findings to evaluate the role of diabetes in patient outcomes. A review for this variable yielded the following results:

		Not healed	Healed
Diabetic	<60 mmHg	6	1
	>60 mmHg	4	12
Nondiabetic	<60 mmHg	9	2
	>60 mmHg	1	15

516. According to these data, which of the following statements is NOT true?

A. A higher percentage of patients with diabetes did not heal.
B. An ankle pressure of > 60 mmHg was a better indication of healing potential than a pressure of < 60 mmHg for both groups.
C. Diabetics with > 60 mmHg ankle pressures that did not heal had calcific arteries causing falsely elevated pressure.
D. About an equal percentage of patients in each group had pressure < 60 mmHg.
E. Healing of a toe amputation site does occur in some patients with pressures < 60 mmHg.

517. In Kappa statistics, if there is no relationship between the two variables being compared, the Kappa value is:

A. Zero
B. 1.00
C. –1.00
D. Greater than 1.00
E. Less than 1.00

518. You are performing a carotid study on a patient who suffers cardiac arrest. You should first immediately:

    A. Administer a precordial thump.
    B. Deliver three mouth-to-mouth breaths.
    C. Administer 15 chest compressions.
    D. Call a code.
    E. Try to find the patient's medications.

519. Your patient begins to fall while getting off the examination table. You should:

    A. Catch him under the arms.
    B. Catch him around the waist.
    C. Let him fall, since you may just hurt him worse by interfering.
    D. Guide the fall, protecting his head.
    E. Start filling out the incident report.

PART VIII

Hall of Images

Duplex Ultrasonography
Pressures & Waveforms
Color Flow Imaging
Angiography

DUPLEX ULTRASONOGRAPHY

520. This image of the internal carotid artery demonstrates:

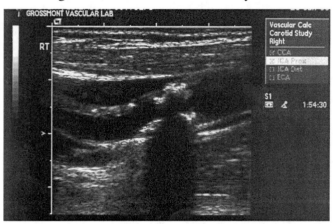

    A. Probable ulceration in the lesion on the deep wall.
    B. Probable ulceration in the lesion on the superficial wall.
    C. Total occlusion, with absence of flow distal to the lesion.
    D. Acoustic shadowing.
    E. A and B.

521. Which statement about this spectral display from the superficial femoral artery is TRUE?

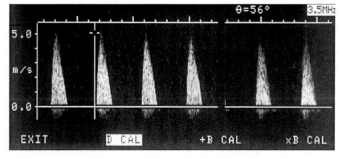

    A. It is within normal limits.

B. It suggests borderline velocity increase, compatible with approximately 50% stenosis.

C. It suggests severe velocity increase, compatible with >75% stenosis.

D. It suggests retrograde flow due to collateralization.

E. It is nondiagnostic.

522. Which statement best describes these waveforms from the common carotid, internal carotid, and external carotid arteries?

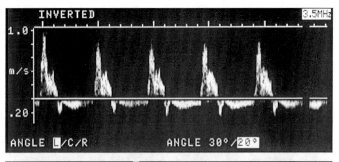

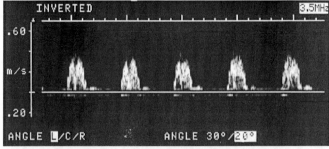

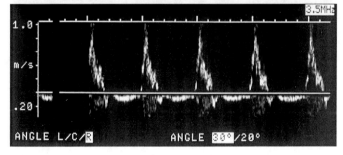

A. They are within normal limits.

B. They suggest common carotid occlusion.

C. They suggest aortic valve stenosis.

D. They suggest aortic valve regurgitation.

E. They suggest contralateral ICA occlusion.

523. This image is from the proximal and distal thigh of a patient a few months following fempop Gore-Tex bypass graft surgery. (The echoes within the graft are from the color flow display, reproduced here in black and white.) Which statement best describes the findings?

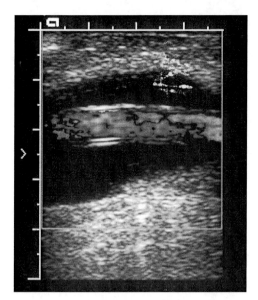

A. They are within normal limits.
B. They suggest deep vein thrombosis.
C. They suggest severe graft stenosis.
D. They suggest graft occlusion.
E. They suggest graft infection.

524. What is represented on this waveform from a left vertebral artery?

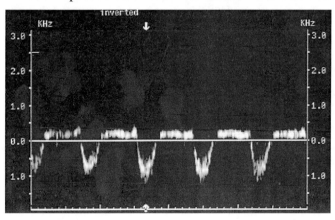

A. It is within normal limits.
B. It suggests transitional vertebral steal.
C. It suggests retrograde flow throughout the cardiac cycle.
D. It suggests severe vertebral stenosis.
E. It is nondiagnostic.

525. In the patient from the previous question, you would expect arm pressures to be:

A. Normal
B. Lower on the right
C. Lower on the left
D. Reduced compared to lower-extremity pressures
E. Immeasurable

526. In this spectral display, the same patient has clenched his fist for three minutes. What effect has the fist clenching had?

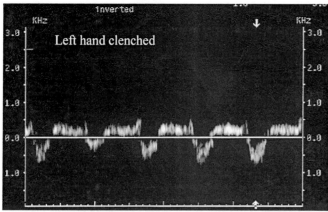

With left hand clenched.

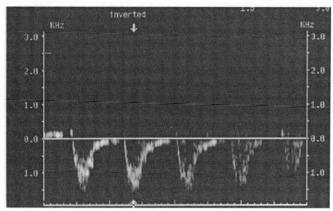

On release of clenching.

A. The exercise causes flow to become retrograde throughout the cardiac cycle.
B. The exercise causes flow to return to antegrade throughout the cardiac cycle.
C. The exercise has no effect on the vertebral artery.
D. The patient will suffer posterior-circulation symptoms.
E. The patient will suffer unilateral visual symptoms.

527. This waveform from an internal carotid artery is measured at > 273 cm/sec peak systolic velocity and 125 cm/sec end-diastolic velocity. It suggests:

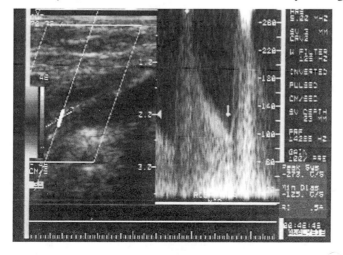

    A. Normal ICA velocities

    B. 30–40% stenosis

    C. Borderline for 50% stenosis

    D. Borderline for 80% stenosis

    E. >90% stenosis

528. This image from the proximal thigh suggests:

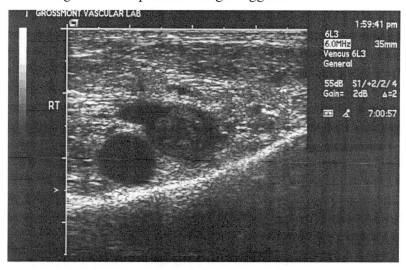

    A. Acute arterial occlusion

    B. Acute venous thrombosis

    C. Chronic peripheral arterial disease

    D. Chronic venous obstruction

    E. Hematoma

529. What is suggested in this spectral display?

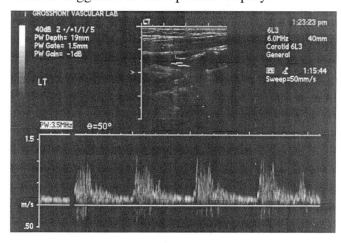

    A. It suggests turbulent flow.

    B. The beam angle suggests that flow is retrograde.

    C. The Doppler beam angle relative to flow is too high for accurate velocity measurement.

    D. The systolic window is clear, suggesting laminar flow.

    E. End-diastolic velocities suggest severe stenosis.

530. This femoral artery waveform demonstrates:

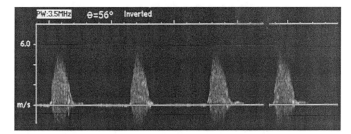

A. Normal velocities and flow character
B. Poor angle correction, precluding accurate velocity estimate
C. Turbulent flow at systole
D. Severely elevated peak-systolic velocities
E. C and D

531. This image is from the carotid bifurcation. It demonstrates:

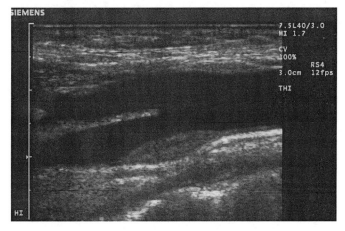

A. Widely patent arteries
B. Heterogeneous plaque that appears to create moderate (<50%) stenosis
C. Homogeneous plaque that appears to create moderate (<50%) stenosis
D. Heterogeneous plaque that appears to create severe (>80%) stenosis
E. Homogeneous plaque that appears to create severe (>80%) stenosis

532. This image was taken just distal to the groin; femoral vessels are seen deep in the field of view. The structure with the measurement cursors represents:

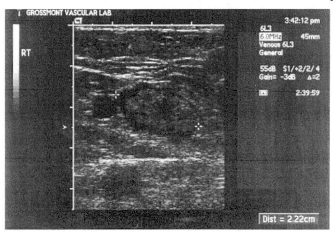

A. Hematoma

B. Highly-vascularized tumor
C. Baker's cyst
D. Pseudoaneurysm
E. Lymph node

533. This image is at the popliteal level and suggests:

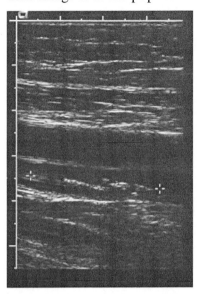

A. Calcific plaque creating arterial occlusion
B. Acute deep vein thrombosis
C. Chronic venous thrombosis
D. Baker's cyst
E. Valve leaflets in the popliteal vein

534. This image from the mid calf suggests:

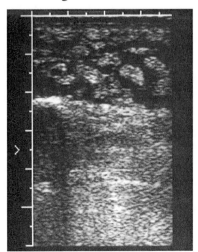

A. Pronounced edema
B. Hematoma
C. Multiple collaterals
D. Pseudoaneurysm
E. Tumor

535. Which disorder is most likely the cause of the condition in the preceding image?

    A. Cellulitis
    B. Chronic arterial obstruction
    C. Acute deep vein thrombosis
    D. Acute arterial occlusion
    E. Trauma

536. This spectral waveform from the distal internal carotid artery suggests:

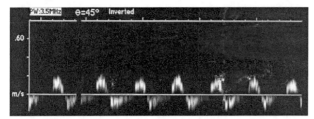

    A. Severe proximal ICA stenosis
    B. Severe common carotid artery stenosis
    C. Occlusion at the ICA origin
    D. Brain death
    E. Postendarterectomy flow changes

537. This internal carotid artery waveform has a peak systolic velocity of 272 cm/sec and an end-diastolic velocity of 88 cm/sec. It is compatible with:

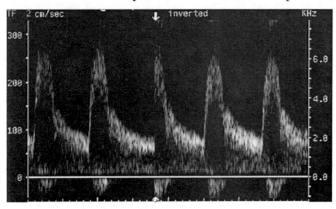

    A. Moderate (<50%) stenosis
    B. Moderately severe (50-80%) stenosis
    C. Severe (>80%) stenosis
    D. Distal total occlusion
    E. The waveform is nondiagnostic

538. In this same patient who has had four episodes of amaurosis fugax in the last week, the most likely course of action would be:

    A. Restudy in six months
    B. Restudy in one month
    C. Immediate angiography
    D. Immediate endarterectomy
    E. Neurological consult

539. This waveform from the origin of the internal carotid artery suggests:

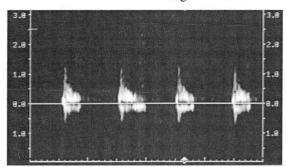

    A. Severe proximal ICA stenosis
    B. Severe common carotid artery stenosis
    C. Occlusion at the ICA origin
    D. Brain death
    E. Postendarterectomy flow changes

540. This waveform is from a right vertebral artery. Which statement is NOT true?

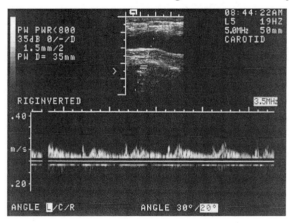

    A. Flow is antegrade.
    B. There is flow during diastole.
    C. The waveform morphology suggests a developing abnormal pressure gradient proximally.
    D. The waveform suggests subclavian or innominate obstruction.
    E. The waveform suggests distal occlusion.

541. This image of the proximal internal carotid artery might suggest:

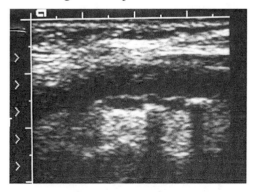

    A. Intraplaque hemorrhage

    B. Minimal homogeneous plaque at the ICA origin
    C. Pronounced calcification
    D. Severe stenosis of ICA origin
    E. ICA occlusion

542. Which of the following describes this image from the common femoral vein?

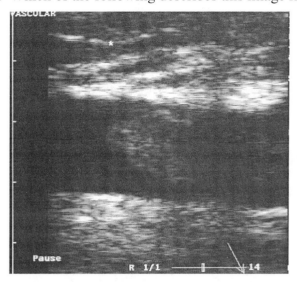

    A. The intraluminal echoes are homogeneous in character.
    B. The intraluminal echoes are heterogeneous in character.
    C. It suggests acute thrombosis.
    D. It suggests chronic thrombosis.
    E. A and C
    F. A and D
    G. B and C
    H. B and D

543. Which of the following statements about this continuous-wave Doppler waveform is
    TRUE?

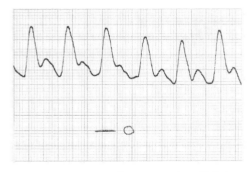

    A. It represents the posterior tibial artery.
    B. It represents the brachial artery.
    C. It is a high-resistance waveform.
    D. It is a low-resistance waveform.
    E. It is proximal to a total occlusion.

544. This CW Doppler waveform is from a posterior tibial artery. The ankle pressure was measured and divided by the higher brachial pressure to arrive at an ankle/arm ratio of 0.56. Which of the following is true?

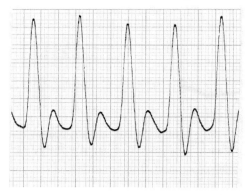

    A. There is something wrong here.
    B. This is within normal limits.

545. This image, from the medial popliteal space of a patient with pain behind the knee and calf edema, most likely suggests:

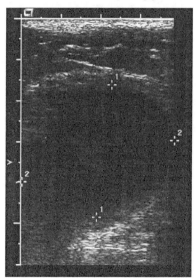

    A. Pseudoaneurysm
    B. Baker's cyst
    C. Popliteal artery aneurysm
    D. Hematoma
    E. Cystic adventitial degeneration

PRESSURES & WAVEFORMS

These waveform-and-pressure cases are somewhat idealized to free them of some of the real-life ambiguities that often show up. Try to apply specific diagnostic criteria to these when deciding what, if anything, is wrong.

Tip on terminology:

Stenosis is narrowing.

Occlusion is total loss of lumen—completely blocked. One can't always be sure which is going on in a waveform-and-pressure study, but there are some mainstream criteria that can sometimes distinguish the two.

Obstruction is a useful word that means either stenosis or occlusion without specifying which.

546. Which of the following describes what is seen on the right lower extremity of patient "Bob"?

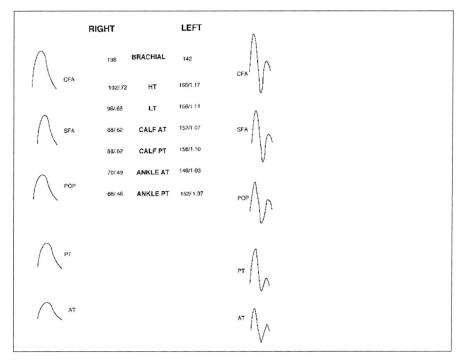

A. Aortoiliac obstruction
B. Iliac occlusion
C. Femoral stenosis
D. Tibial obstruction
E. Within normal limits

547. Which of the following describes what is seen on the left lower extremity of patient "Bob"?

A. Aortoiliac obstruction
B. Iliac obstruction
C. Femoral obstruction
D. Tibial obstruction
E. Within normal limits

548. Which of the following describes what is seen on the right lower extremity of patient "Myra"?

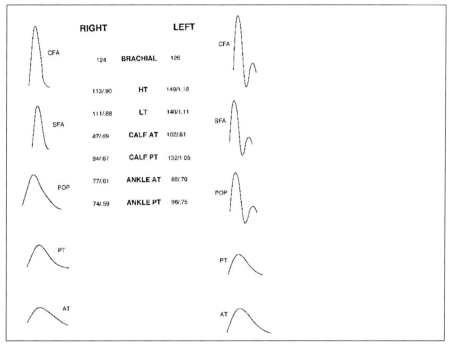

RIGHT		LEFT
124	BRACHIAL	126
113/.90	HT	149/1.18
111/.88	LT	140/1.11
87/.69	CALF AT	102/.81
84/.67	CALF PT	132/1.05
77/.61	ANKLE AT	88/.70
74/.59	ANKLE PT	96/.75

A. Aortoiliac obstruction
B. Iliac stenosis
C. Femoral stenosis
D. Tibial stenosis
E. Within normal limits

549. What is on the left lower extremity of patient "Myra"?

A. Distal femoral stenosis
B. Popliteal stenosis
C. Proximal posterior tibial stenosis and mid anterior tibial stenosis
D. Mid posterior tibial stenosis and proximal anterior tibial stenosis
E. Proximal posterior tibial and anterior tibial stenosis

The nine color plates that appear on the following pages apply to questions 550–560.

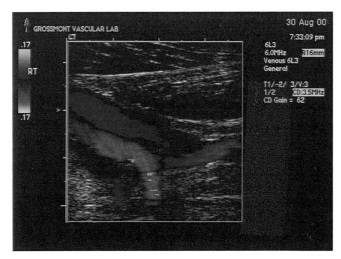

Color Plate 1. See questions 550 and 551.

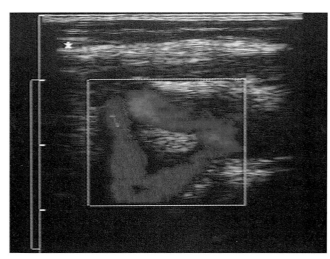

Color Plate 4. See question 554.

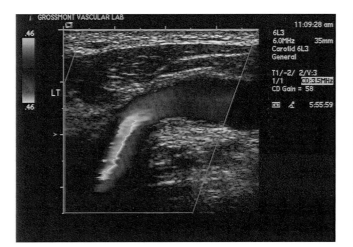

Color Plate 2. See question 552.

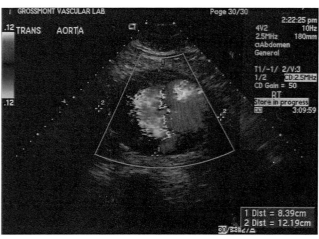

Color Plate 5. See questions 555 and 556.

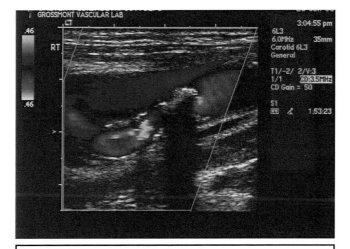

Color Plate 3 (above). See question 553.
Color Plate 6 (right). See question 557.

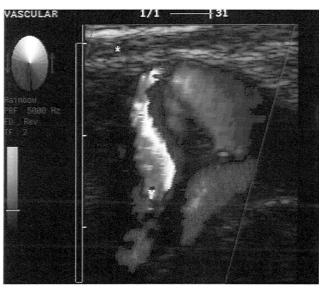

REGISTRY 101

Test-Taking Tips from the Preface

Read each question twice before answering. Guess how easy it is to get one word wrong and blow it.

Try to answer the question before looking at the choices. Formulating an answer before peeking at the possibilities minimizes the distractibility of the incorrect answer choices, which in the test-making business are called— guess what!—*distractors*.

Knock off the easy ones first. First answer the easy questions. Then go back for the more difficult items. Next attack the really tough ones. Taking notes on long or tricky questions can jog your memory or put the question in new light.

Guessing. Passing the exam depends on the number of correct answers you make. Because unanswered questions are counted as *in*correct, it makes sense to guess when all else fails. The ARDMS itself advises that "it is to the candidate's advantage to answer all possible questions." Guessing alone improves your chances of scoring a point from 0 (for an unanswered question) to 20% (for randomly picking one of five possible answers). Eliminating answer choices you know or suspect are wrong further improves your odds of success. By using your knowledge and skill to eliminate three of the five answer choices before guessing, for example, you increase your odds of scoring a point to 50%.

Don't second-guess. Actual studies indicate that when you return to a question and change the answer, you'll probably be wrong. Change an answer only if you're quite sure.

Pace yourself; watch the time. Work methodically and quickly to answer those you know, and make your best guesses at the gnarly ones. Leave no question unanswered.

Don't despair 50 minutes into the exam. At some point you may feel that things just aren't going well. Take 10 seconds to breathe deeply and relax. You need only about three out of four correct answers to pass. If you've prepared reasonably well you can do it, even with sweat running down your back.

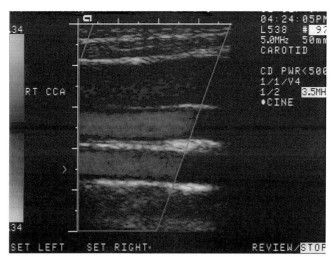

Color Plate 7. See question 558.

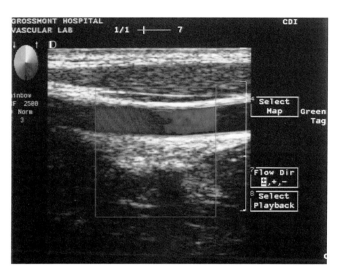

Color Plate 8. See question 559.

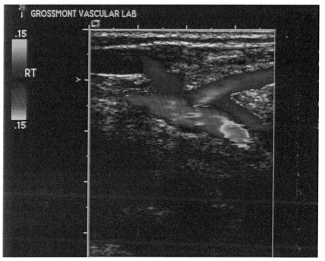

Color Plate 9. See question 560.

COLOR FLOW IMAGING

The following questions refer to the color plates that appear on the previous pages. Several of these questions are meant to be a tad confusing at first. This is to cultivate a healthy suspicion of color displays, as they can lead you astray if you jump to conclusions. Besides, that extra modality costs your institution a lot; you've got to have some fun with it.

550. The image in Color Plate 1 on the previous pages represents the popliteal artery bifurcating into its branches, taken from a posteromedial approach just distal to the popliteal space. (In the image, the distal popliteal vein lies just superficial to the artery, with its cephalad flow shown in blue.) The branch going vertical/deep in the center is the:

    A. Posterior tibial artery
    B. Anterior tibial artery
    C. Peroneal artery
    D. Tibioperoneal trunk
    E. Supreme genicular artery

551. In Color Plate 1 the tibioperoneal trunk artery is:

    A. Demonstrating retrograde flow due to collateralization
    B. Demonstrating aliasing, suggesting greatly increased velocities
    C. Demonstrating antegrade flow
    D. Demonstrating absence of flow due to occlusion
    E. Not visible in this image

552. Color Plate 2 represents the internal carotid artery, with the color flow demonstrating:

    A. Flow reversal due to pronounced stenosis
    B. Aliasing, suggesting increased velocities due to stenosis
    C. Aliasing, suggesting increased velocities due to flow running downhill
    D. Aliasing caused by changing frequency shifts
    E. Blunted flow due to distal occlusion

553. The internal carotid artery in Color Plate 3 demonstrates:

    A. Interruption of the color flow due to acoustic shadowing
    B. ICA occlusion with reconstitution via ophthalmic artery collateralization
    C. ICA occlusion with reconstitution via circle of Willis collateralization
    D. Extrinsic compression of the ICA
    E. Probable carotid body tumor

554. The image in Color Plate 4 is from the carotid bifurcation, with the distal common carotid artery just visible at the right of the color box. The superficial branch is the internal carotid artery. Which of the following is TRUE?

    A. The flow in the superficial branch is retrograde.
    B. The flow in the deeper branch is retrograde.
    C. The vertical segment is the internal carotid artery.

D. The vertical segment is the external carotid artery.

E. A and C.

555. Color Plate 5 is a transverse image from the abdominal aorta. It demonstrates:

A. The right/left iliac bifurcation

B. The inferior vena cava to the left of the aorta

C. Renal artery stenosis

D. Normal multiphasic flow

E. A large aneurysm

556. In the same transverse aortic image (Color Plate 5), which is NOT true?

A. Incomplete filling is due to mural thrombus.

B. This patient would probably be considered for surgery.

C. The diameter is larger than 5 cm.

D. This is the preferred plane for diameter measurement.

E. This is probably from a level inferior to the renal arteries.

557. The tortuous internal carotid artery in Color Plate 6 demonstrates:

A. The French tricolor

B. Helical flow pattern beyond the tortuosity

C. Faster flow along the outer wall (at left)

D. Aliasing

E. All of the above

558. The image in Color Plate 7 was taken from a supraclavicular approach with the beam aimed inferiorly. Which of the following correctly describes the image?

A. This patient has the common anatomic variant of double subclavian arteries.

B. This patient has retrograde flow in an accessory subclavian vein.

C. This is an artifactual image.

D. This patient has the common anatomic variant of double subclavian veins.

E. There is pronounced aliasing in the artery.

559. The image in Color Plate 8 demonstrates normal flow in the common carotid artery. This statement is:

A. True

B. False

560. In the image of a radial/ulnar artery bifurcation that appears in Color Plate 9, the ulnar artery, as usual, dives deeper in the field. Which of the following statements are true?

1. The radial artery flow is antegrade.
2. The radial artery flow is retrograde.
3. The brachial artery flow is antegrade.
4. The brachial artery flow is retrograde.
5. The ulnar artery flow is antegrade.
6. The ulnar artery flow is retrograde.

A. 1, 3, and 5
B. 1, 3, and 6
C. 2, 3, and 5
D. 2, 3, and 6
E. 2, 4, and 6

ANGIOGRAPHY

561. This angiogram suggests:

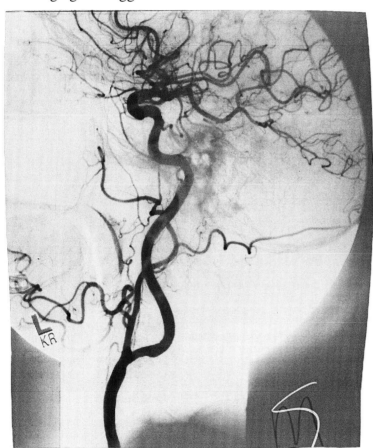

A. Normal carotid bifurcation
B. Moderate ICA stenosis
C. Severe ICA stenosis
D. Total occlusion of ICA
E. It is nondiagnostic

562. The arrow in the same angiogram is pointing to:

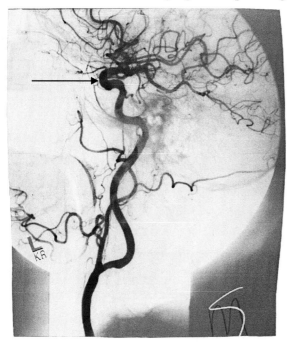

A. The anterior cerebral artery
B. The posterior cerebral artery
C. The ophthalmic artery
D. The external carotid artery
E. The internal carotid artery

563. This lower extremity angiogram demonstrates:

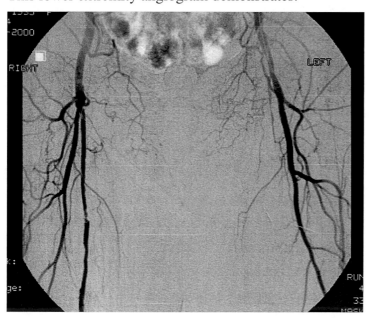

A. Severe SFA stenosis on the right
B. Severe SFA stenosis on the left
C. Severe CFA stenosis on the right
D. Severe CFA stenosis on the left

E. No significant femoral artery stenosis

564. Which of the following statements about this angiogram is FALSE?

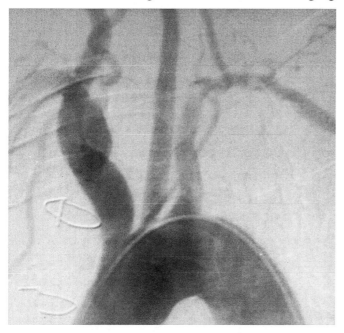

A. The middle branch is the left common carotid artery.
B. There is vessel overlap at the innominate bifurcation.
C. The vertebral arteries are visible taking off from the subclavian arteries.
D. The catheter is visible in the aortic arch.
E. There is high-grade stenosis of the left subclavian artery.

565. This angiogram demonstrates:

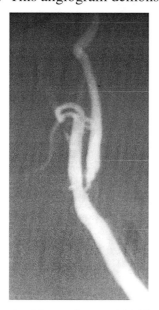

A. Normal carotid bifurcation
B. Moderate ICA stenosis
C. Severe ICA stenosis
D. Total occlusion of ICA

E. It is nondiagnostic.

566. The arrow is pointing to:

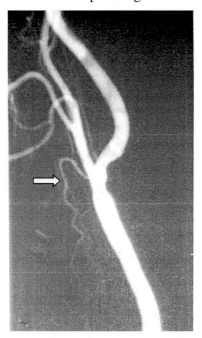

A. The superficial temporal artery
B. The facial artery
C. The superior thyroid artery
D. The angular artery
E. The vertebral artery

567. The angiogram in the previous question suggests:

A. Normal carotid bifurcation
B. Moderate ICA stenosis
C. Severe ICA stenosis
D. Total occlusion of ICA
E. It is nondiagnostic.

568. This rather busy angiogram demonstrates:

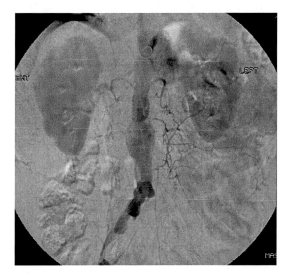

A. Aortic stenosis, right iliac occlusion, and left iliac stenosis
B. Aortic stenosis, left iliac occlusion, and right iliac stenosis
C. Aortic aneurysm, right iliac occlusion, and left iliac stenosis
D. Aortic aneurysm, left iliac occlusion, and right iliac stenosis
E. Aortic occlusion with multiple collaterals reconstituting the iliacs

569. This lower extremity angiogram demonstrates occlusion of:

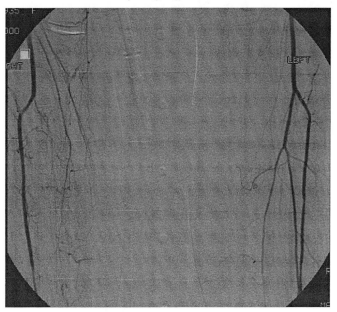

A. Right anterior tibial artery
B. Left anterior tibial artery
C. Right tibioperoneal artery
D. Left tibioperoneal artery
E. Right popliteal artery

570. This carotid angiogram demonstrates:

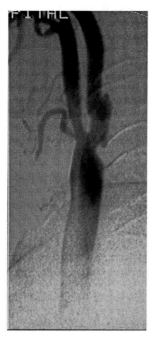

A. Normal carotid bifurcation
B. Preocclusive (>90%) ICA and ECA stenosis
C. Moderate stenosis of ICA and ECA with probable ulceration
D. Significant ECA stenosis and normal ICA
E. ECA occlusion and moderate ICA stenosis

571. This carotid angiogram demonstrates:

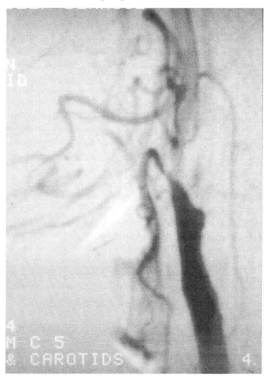

A. ECA occlusion and moderate ICA stenosis
B. ICA occlusion and severe ECA stenosis
C. Severe stenosis of ICA and ECA

D. Occlusion of common carotid artery

E. The image is nondiagnostic

572. This lower extremity angiogram demonstrates:

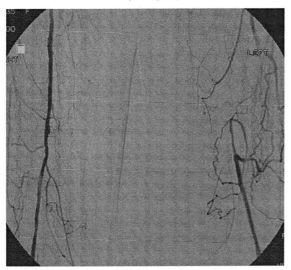

A. Occlusion of the right superficial femoral artery with distal reconstitution

B. Occlusion of the left superficial femoral artery with distal reconstitution

C. Severe stenosis of the right superficial femoral artery

D. Severe stenosis of the left superficial femoral artery

E. Severe trifurcation disease

573. This angiogram is taken in AP (anteroposterior) view. It represents:

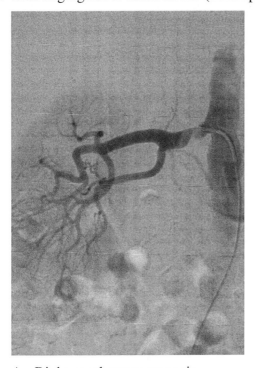

A. Right renal artery stenosis

B. Right renal artery occlusion

C. Left renal artery stenosis

    D. Left renal artery occlusion

    E. Hypoplastic inferior mesenteric artery

574. This angiogram demonstrates:

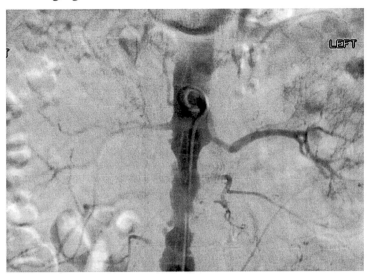

    A. Abdominal aortic aneurysm with mural thrombus

    B. Abdominal aortic occlusion with multiple collaterals

    C. Abdominal aortic stenosis

    D. Superior mesenteric artery occlusion

    E. Double left renal arteries

575. This angiogram demonstrates:

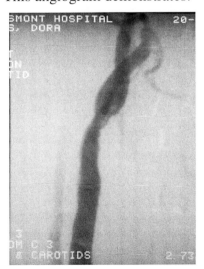

    A. Vessel overlap, making diagnosis difficult

    B. Moderate ICA stenosis

    C. Severe ICA stenosis

    D. Total occlusion of ICA

    E. Filling defect, suggesting total occlusion of the external branch

PART IX

Answers, Explanations & References

Anatomy, Physiology & Hemodynamics
Cerebrovascular Disease
Venous Disease
Peripheral Arterial Disease
Abdominal & Visceral Vascular Disease
Miscellaneous Conditions & Tests
Hall of Images

ANATOMY, PHYSIOLOGY & FLUID DYNAMICS

1.   D. The innominate artery.

   The innominate artery (also called the brachiocephalic trunk) is the first of the three great vessels to arise from the aorta.

   ▷Rumwell CB, McPharlin M: *Vascular Technology: An Illustrated Review*, 5th edition. Pasadena, CA, Davies Publishing, 2015, p 3.

   ▷Belanger A: *Vascular Anatomy and Physiology*. Pasadena, CA, Davies Publishing, 1999, p 53.

2.   B. Superior thyroid.

   The superior thyroid artery is usually the first branch of the external carotid artery. "Internal mammary" is another name for the "internal thoracic" artery.

   ▷Rumwell CB, McPharlin M: *Vascular Technology: An Illustrated Review*, 5th edition. Pasadena, CA, Davies Publishing, 2015, p 200.

3.   E. Facial artery.

   The facial artery terminates as the angular artery.

   ▷Rumwell CB, McPharlin M: *Vascular Technology: An Illustrated Review*, 5th edition. Pasadena, CA, Davies Publishing, 2015, p 200.

▷Belanger A: *Vascular Anatomy and Physiology*. Pasadena,
CA, Davies Publishing, 1999, p 77.

4.   C. Superficial temporal.

The superficial temporal artery is the terminal branch off the external carotid.

▷Belanger A: *Vascular Anatomy and Physiology*. Pasadena,
CA, Davies Publishing, 1999, p 79.

5.   C. Thyroid cartilage.

*The external and internal carotid arteries are formed from the common carotid artery,
usually at the upper border of the thyroid cartilage.*

▷Belanger A: *Vascular Anatomy and Physiology*. Pasadena,
CA, Davies Publishing, 1999, p 73.

6.   B. Superior thyroid artery.

▷Rumwell CB, McPharlin M: *Vascular Technology: An
Illustrated Review*, 5th edition. Pasadena, CA, Davies
Publishing, 2015, p 200.

▷Belanger A: *Vascular Anatomy and Physiology*. Pasadena,
CA, Davies Publishing, 1999, pp 71–97.

7.   D. Middle communicating artery.

There are only the anterior and posterior communicating arteries.

▷Belanger A: *Vascular Anatomy and Physiology*. Pasadena,
CA, Davies Publishing, 1999, p 86.

8.   E. All of the above.

*The external carotid artery has eight branches. The following four branches arise in the
carotid triangle: the superior thyroid, lingual, facial, and the ascending pharyngeal
arteries.*

▷Rumwell CB, McPharlin M: *Vascular Technology: An
Illustrated Review*, 5th edition. Pasadena, CA, Davies
Publishing, 2015, p 200.

9.   B. Thyroid cartilage.

*The thyroid cartilage forms a prominence that is especially visible in tall, thin, socially
awkward males.*

▷Belanger A: *Vascular Anatomy and Physiology*. Pasadena,
CA, Davies Publishing, 1999, p 73.

10.   A. The subclavian artery.

The vertebral artery arises from the dorsosuperior aspect of the ascending (first) portion of the subclavian artery. A not-uncommon variant is the vertebral artery arising directly from the aortic arch.

▷Rumwell CB, McPharlin M: *Vascular Technology: An Illustrated Review*, 5th edition. Pasadena, CA, Davies Publishing, 2015, p 201.

11.   A. Maxillary artery.

The infraorbital artery is a terminal branch of the maxillary artery. It creates one of the potential anastomoses with orbital branches that can provide collateral pathways in the event of carotid obstruction.

▷Belanger A: *Vascular Anatomy and Physiology*. Pasadena, CA, Davies Publishing, 1999, p 79.

12.   C. Basilar artery.

This system is called the vertebrobasilar system and is responsible for the circulation to the posterior portion of the brain.

▷Rumwell CB, McPharlin M: *Vascular Technology: An Illustrated Review*, 5th edition. Pasadena, CA, Davies Publishing, 2015, p 202.

13.   D. Ophthalmic artery.

Even though there is often a branch called the caroticotympanic artery, the ophthalmic artery is regarded as the first major branch of the internal carotid artery. It is central to indirect physiological testing.

▷Rumwell CB, McPharlin M: *Vascular Technology: An Illustrated Review*, 5th edition. Pasadena, CA, Davies Publishing, 2015, p 199.

14.   D. Carotid and vertebral arteries.

This remarkable connection of the carotid and vertebral arteries—illustrated below— makes possible the ability of the brain to withstand (sometimes) extracranial carotid occlusion without significant symptoms.

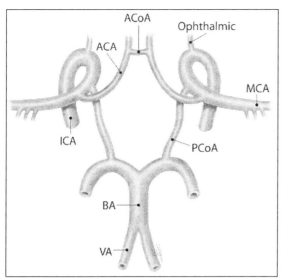

Drawing by Denise Eggman. Used with permission.

▷Rumwell CB, McPharlin M: *Vascular Technology: An Illustrated Review*, 5th edition. Pasadena, CA, Davies Publishing, 2015, p 201.

15. B. Nasal, frontal, and supraorbital arteries.

These branches are assessed in the periorbital Doppler examination for carotid artery disease. Questions about periorbital Doppler assessment are no longer included on the ARDMS exam.

▷Rumwell CB, McPharlin M: *Vascular Technology: An Illustrated Review*, 5th edition. Pasadena, CA, Davies Publishing, 2015, p 203.

16. C. Superficial temporal and facial arteries.

The supraorbital, frontal, and ophthalmic arteries are all fed by the internal carotid. The vertebral artery is part of the posterior circulation.

▷Rumwell CB, McPharlin M: *Vascular Technology: An Illustrated Review*, 5th edition. Pasadena, CA, Davies Publishing, 2015, p 200.

17. C. Superficial temporal artery.

The superficial temporal artery is not an intracranial vessel. Leptomeningeal collaterals and the rete mirable ("wonderful net") are potential collateral pathways of lesser importance than the circle of Willis arteries.

▷Rumwell CB, McPharlin M: *Vascular Technology: An Illustrated Review*, 5th edition. Pasadena, CA, Davies Publishing, 2015, p 203.

▷Pellerito JS, Polak JF: *Introduction to Vascular Ultrasonography*, 6th edition. Philadelphia, Elsevier Saunders, 2012, pp 231–243.

18.   B. This statement about the internal carotid artery—"It supplies a high-resistance system"—is false.

The internal carotid artery feeds a low-resistance system.

▷Rumwell CB, McPharlin M: *Vascular Technology: An Illustrated Review*, 5th edition. Pasadena, CA, Davies Publishing, 2015, pp 199, 228.

19.   D. Middle cerebral and anterior cerebral arteries.

At a depth of approximately 60 mm, the internal carotid artery at its distal limit bifurcates into the middle cerebral and anterior cerebral arteries. Flow in the MCA is toward the Doppler beam, while flow in the ACA is away from the beam. The TCD sample volume is fairly large, so both arteries appear on the spectral display, above and below baseline, and the question specifies a bidirectional waveform. The MCA/ACA bifurcation waveform is a common reference point that helps the practitioner of blind TCD (i.e., non-duplex) to be sure of orientation and identification).

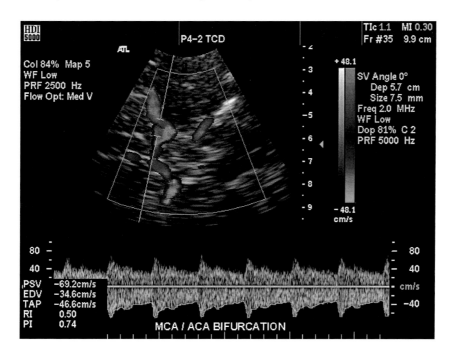

Choice A seems possibly correct and includes PCA and ACA. Both can be seen through the transtemporal window at 60 mm depth and the PCA is antegrade flow and ACA is retrograde flow. In a normal circle of Willis, though, you're extremely unlikely to get both PCA and ACA in the same sample volume (see illustration with explanation to question 14 above). Choice B is incorrect because you can only visualize the vertebrals through the transforaminal window, and choice E is incorrect because they are two separate vessels visualized in two separate windows.

▷Rumwell CB, McPharlin M: *Vascular Technology: An Illustrated Review*, 5th edition. Pasadena, CA, Davies Publishing, 2015, p 244.

20. D. Absence or hypoplasia of one or both of the communicating arteries.

21. D. A. (2); B. (5); C. (1); D. (3); E. (4).

   ▷Belanger A: *Vascular Anatomy and Physiology*. Pasadena,
   CA, Davies Publishing, 1999, pp 49–97.

22. A. Normal flow dynamics.

   *Flow separation at the posterior wall of the carotid bulb occurs because the linear
   momentum of the flow is disrupted by the large sinus and sharp curve at the carotid bulb.
   Flow separation depends on a relatively disease-free bulb.*

   ▷Rumwell CB, McPharlin M: *Vascular Technology: An
   Illustrated Review*, 5th edition. Pasadena, CA, Davies
   Publishing, 2015, p 26.

   ▷Ku DN, Lumsden A: Blood flow patterns in cerebrovascular
   disease. In Bernstein EF (ed): *Noninvasive Diagnostic
   Techniques in Vascular Disease*. St. Louis, Mosby, 1985, pp
   73–83.

23. A. A common origin of the innominate and left common carotid arteries.

   *A common origin of the innominate and left common carotid arteries is by far the most
   common variant anatomy of the aortic arch, occurring in approximately 22% of
   individuals.*

   ▷Kadir S: Regional anatomy of the thoracic aorta. In *Atlas of
   Normal and Variant Angiographic Anatomy*. Philadelphia,
   Saunders, 1991, pp 19–54.

24. E. All are correct.

   *The great saphenous vein passes upward on the anteromedial calf and the posteromedial to
   medial thigh. It ends by passing through the saphenous hiatus in the deep fascia of the
   proximal thigh to enter the common femoral vein.*

   ▷Rumwell CB, McPharlin M: *Vascular Technology: An
   Illustrated Review*, 5th edition. Pasadena, CA, Davies
   Publishing, 2015, p 270.

   ▷Belanger A: *Vascular Anatomy and Physiology*. Pasadena,
   CA, Davies Publishing, 1999, p 109.

25. A. This statement about the saphenous vein—"It passes superiorly on the lateral side of the
    knee"—is NOT correct.

   ▷Rumwell CB, McPharlin M: *Vascular Technology: An
   Illustrated Review*, 5th edition. Pasadena, CA, Davies
   Publishing, 2015, p 270.

   ▷Belanger A: *Vascular Anatomy and Physiology*. Pasadena,
   CA, Davies Publishing, 1999, p 109.

26. B. Posterior arch vein.

The posterior accessory vein (formerly "posterior arch vein"), since it connects the Cockett perforators in the calf, is implicated in the formation of venous stasis ulcers.

The International Union of Phlebology (IUP) issued guidelines for venous nomenclature in 2003. Many of the recommendations have been slow to gain favor, but we should be good citizens and try to get standardized. These are important changes for us, since we examine these veins frequently. As the right-hand column says, avoid the old nomenclature, but be prepared to hear and read the old terms fairly often. Be ready both ways.

New IUP LE vein nomenclature	Old nomenclature—avoid, but be ready to hear/read
Femoral vein	Superficial femoral vein
Great saphenous (GSV)	Greater saphenous, long saphenous
Small saphenous (SSV)	Lesser saphenous
Posterior tibial perforators Lower, middle, upper	Cockett perforators I, II, III
Paratibial perforators	Boyd's perforator(s)
Femoral canal perforators	Dodd's and/or Hunterian perforators
Posterior accessory vein (of the leg)	Posterior arch vein

▷Rumwell CB, McPharlin M: *Vascular Technology: An Illustrated Review*, 5th edition. Pasadena, CA, Davies Publishing, 2015, p 271.

▷Gloviczhi P, Rhodes JM: Management of perforator vein incompetence. In Rutherford RB (ed): *Vascular Surgery*, 5th edition. Philadelphia, Saunders, 2000, p 2022.

27. E. Below the knee.

Good information on the perforators is not easy to find; see Bergan in the reference list. A quick review:

There are many, many perforating veins (veins that penetrate the deep fascia that covers the muscles of the leg, sending flow from superficial veins to deep veins). The main ones are the posterior-tibial perforators in the mid to distal calf (again, connected by the posterior accessory saphenous vein), paratibial perforators below the medial knee, femoral canal perforators around mid to distal thigh. See the illustration. And check again with the table above regarding proper nomenclature.

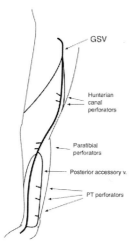

▷Bergan J (ed): *The Vein Book.* St. Louis, Elsevier Academic Press, 2007.

▷Gloviczhi P, Rhodes JM: Management of perforator vein incompetence. In Rutherford RB (ed): *Vascular Surgery*, 5th edition. Philadelphia, Saunders, 2000, p 2022.

28. D. Crosses posterior to the right common iliac artery just distal to the aortic bifurcation.

    The left common iliac vein is medial to the artery. The vena cava is to the right of the aorta. Thus, the left venous system must cross some arterial structure to communicate with the vena cava. Answer D is the usual anatomic relationship.

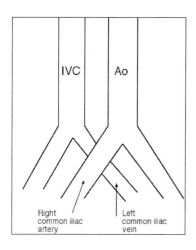

▷Pellerito JS, Polak JF: *Introduction to Vascular Ultrasonography*, 6th edition. Philadelphia, Elsevier Saunders, 2012, pp 368–371.

29. C. Great saphenous vein, femoral vein, profunda femoris vein.

    ▷Ridgway DA: *Introduction to Vascular Scanning*, 4th edition. Pasadena, CA, Davies Publishing, 2014, pp 197, 206–208.

30. A. Ulnar and radial veins to the axillary vein.

▷Rumwell CB, McPharlin M: *Vascular Technology: An Illustrated Review*, 5th edition. Pasadena, CA, Davies Publishing, 2015, p 272.

31. C. Distal deep femoral vein.

Because of its depth, the distal deep femoral vein is usually very difficult to image.

▷Pellerito JS, Polak JF: *Introduction to Vascular Ultrasonography*, 6th edition. Philadelphia, Elsevier Saunders, 2012, p 363.

32. C. The calf muscles.

The term "muscle pump" refers to the mechanism of venous return from the lower extremities, which must overcome significant hydrostatic pressure in the upright patient. The veins and sinuses fill during relaxation; then contraction of lower extremity muscles propels blood cephalad.

▷Rumwell CB, McPharlin M: *Vascular Technology: An Illustrated Review*, 5th edition. Pasadena, CA, Davies Publishing, 2015, pp 278–279.

33. E.

34. C.

35. E.

36. B.

Be sure that you can identify also the tibia, the soleal septum, the peroneal vessels, the anterior tibial vessels, and the great saphenous vein. Which aspect is anterior and which is lateral?

▷Pellerito JS, Polak JF: *Introduction to Vascular Ultrasonography*, 6th edition. Philadelphia, Elsevier Saunders, 2012, p 367–369.

▷Talbot SR: Venous imaging technique. In Talbot SR, Oliver MA: *Techniques of Venous Imaging.* Pasadena, CA, Davies Publishing, 1992, p 97.

▷Ridgway DA: *Introduction to Vascular Scanning*, 4th edition. Pasadena, CA, Davies Publishing, 2014, pp 222–224.

37. B. Median cubital vein.

38. B. Cephalic vein.

The deep veins of the upper extremity include the deep palmar venous arch, radial veins, ulnar veins and interosseous veins of the forearm, brachial veins, and axillary vein. The deep veins accompany the same named arteries and are usually paired. The cephalic,

basilic, and median cubital veins are superficial veins. They do not accompany an artery and are not paired.

▷Rumwell CB, McPharlin M: *Vascular Technology: An Illustrated Review*, 5th edition. Pasadena, CA, Davies Publishing, 2015, pp 273, 317.

39. C. On both the right and left sides.

The venous anatomy in the upper torso differs from the arterial anatomy. There are right and left brachiocephalic veins, which receive flow from the internal jugular and subclavian veins, but there is just the right innominate (also called brachiocephalic) artery.

40. D. Basilic vein.

The basilic vein is a superficial vein of the upper extremity that joins with the brachial veins to form the axillary vein. It begins on the ulnar side of the forearm and crosses ventrally at the antecubital region. The basilic vein lies medial to the brachial artery in the upper arm.

▷Rumwell CB, McPharlin M: *Vascular Technology: An Illustrated Review*, 5th edition. Pasadena, CA, Davies Publishing, 2015, pp 273, 317.

41. D. Gastrocnemius veins.

Gastrocnemius veins are commonly seen on the venous duplex scan and may be thrombosed like other calf veins. They should be distinguished from soleal sinuses, which empty into the posterior tibial and peroneal veins in the calf itself.

▷Pellerito JS, Polak JF: *Introduction to Vascular Ultrasonography*, 6th edition. Philadelphia, Elsevier Saunders, 2012, pp 366–367.

42. E. Thinner adventitia and media.

Intimal linings are the same size in arteries and veins—a layer of endothelial cells.

▷Rumwell CB, McPharlin M: *Vascular Technology: An Illustrated Review*, 5th edition. Pasadena, CA, Davies Publishing, 2015, p 13.

43. D. This statement about venous valves—"Allow flow only away from the heart"—is false.

Valves (when they are working properly) allow flow only toward the heart.

▷Rumwell CB, McPharlin M: *Vascular Technology: An Illustrated Review*, 5th edition. Pasadena, CA, Davies Publishing, 2015, p 276.

44. E. Greater length, smaller diameter, and higher blood viscosity.

Poiseuille's resistance equation demonstrates the influences on resistance of length, viscosity, and (inversely and powerfully) radius:

$$R = 8\eta L \div \pi r^4$$

▷Rumwell CB, McPharlin M: *Vascular Technology: An Illustrated Review*, 5th edition. Pasadena, CA, Davies Publishing, 2015, p 21.

45. C. Internal carotid, postprandial superior mesenteric, and renal arteries.

Postprandial (after a meal) superior mesenteric flows have lower resistance, higher diastolic flow character.

▷Rumwell CB, McPharlin M: *Vascular Technology: An Illustrated Review*, 5th edition. Pasadena, CA, Davies Publishing, 2015, pp 28–29.

46. D. This statement about the dorsalis pedis artery—"It is a branch of the peroneal artery"—is NOT correct.

The dorsalis pedis artery continues the anterior tibial artery to the pedal arch.

▷Rumwell CB, McPharlin M: *Vascular Technology: An Illustrated Review*, 5th edition. Pasadena, CA, Davies Publishing, 2015, pp 9–10.

47. D. Inferior vesicle artery.

▷Pellerito JS, Polak JF: *Introduction to Vascular Ultrasonography*, 6th edition. Philadelphia, Elsevier Saunders, 2012, pp 569–572.

48. D. The circumflex.

There are several "circumflex" arteries, some near or proximal to the groin.

▷Belanger A: *Vascular Anatomy and Physiology*. Pasadena, CA, Davies Publishing, 1999, p 67.

49. A. Posterolateral to the superficial femoral artery.

"Profunda femoris" is Latin for "deep femoral," and the two are used interchangeably; thus, the profunda femoris artery is posterior (deep) to the superficial femoral artery. It usually branches posterolateral to the superficial femoral artery (heading toward the femur).

▷Pellerito JS, Polak JF: *Introduction to Vascular Ultrasonography*, 6th edition. Philadelphia, Elsevier Saunders, 2012, p 238.

50. E. Anterior tibial and tibioperoneal trunk; then posterior tibial and peroneal.

▷Rumwell CB, McPharlin M: *Vascular Technology: An Illustrated Review*, 5th edition. Pasadena, CA, Davies Publishing, 2015, p 11.

51. E. Brachial artery to the subclavian artery.

▷Belanger A: *Vascular Anatomy and Physiology*. Pasadena, CA, Davies Publishing, 1999, p 55.

52. B. Right subclavian artery.

The right subclavian artery arises from the innominate artery (brachiocephalic trunk). Obviously this question assumes normal anatomy; there are frequent variants with the brachiocephalic arteries.

▷Belanger A: *Vascular Anatomy and Physiology*. Pasadena, CA, Davies Publishing, 1999, p 53.

53. C. Common femoral artery.

54. C. External iliac artery.

55. A. Laterally.

From the lateral aspect. The right renal artery is usually anterolateral, the left renal usually posterolateral.

▷Pellerito JS, Polak JF: *Introduction to Vascular Ultrasonography*, 6th edition. Philadelphia, Elsevier Saunders, 2012, p 447.

56. A. Crosses anterior to the aorta inferior to the left renal artery.

The aorta is to the left of midline, while the vena cava is to the right. Thus, structures located in the left side of the abdomen must have their venous outflow across the aorta. The left renal vein is anterior to the aorta, usually just inferior to the level of the renal artery.

▷Pellerito JS, Polak JF: *Introduction to Vascular Ultrasonography*, 6th edition. Philadelphia, Elsevier Saunders, 2012, pp 447–448.

57. C. The left renal vein.

The left renal vein travels anterior to the aorta to reach across to the inferior vena cava.

▷Pellerito JS, Polak JF: *Introduction to Vascular Ultrasonography*, 6th edition. Philadelphia, Elsevier Saunders, 2012, p 447.

58. A. The aorta between the celiac trunk and the renal arteries.

The superior mesenteric artery may originate from the celiac trunk.

▷Rumwell CB, McPharlin M: *Vascular Technology: An Illustrated Review*, 5th edition. Pasadena, CA, Davies Publishing, 2015, p 9.

▷Belanger A: *Vascular Anatomy and Physiology*. Pasadena, CA, Davies Publishing, 1999, PP 49–69.

59.   D. Right and left brachiocephalic veins.

Also called the right and left innominate veins. The brachiocephalic vein turns into the subclavian vein at the junction of the internal jugular vein.

▷Belanger A: *Vascular Anatomy and Physiology*. Pasadena, CA, Davies Publishing, 1999, p 103.

60.   C. Superior mesenteric and splenic veins.

The inferior mesenteric vein joins with the splenic vein, which in turn joins with the superior mesenteric vein to become the portal vein.

▷Pellerito JS, Polak JF: *Introduction to Vascular Ultrasonography*, 6th edition. Philadelphia, Elsevier Saunders, 2012, pp 443–444.

61.   A. Superior mesenteric artery.

The renal—artery origins lie just distal to the origin of the superior mesenteric artery (SMA) from the aorta. The left renal vein, which passes across to the inferior vena cava under the proximal SMA and lies anterior and a bit distal to the renal arteries, can also be a useful landmark.

▷Pellerito JS, Polak JF: *Introduction to Vascular Ultrasonography*, 6th edition. Philadelphia, Elsevier Saunders, 2012, p 447.

62.   D. Celiac trunk.

The celiac is the first major branch of the abdominal aorta. It divides into the common hepatic, splenic, and left gastric arteries.

63.   B. Multiple renal arteries.

Multiple renal arteries are the most common anatomic variant of the renal arteries, occurring in as many as 30% of individuals. Multiple renal arteries may occur unilaterally or bilaterally, and they occur with equal frequency on both the right and left sides. They most commonly originate from the abdominal aorta or common iliac arteries but may arise from the superior and inferior mesenteric, median sacral, intercostal, lumbar, adrenal, inferior French, right hepatic, or right colic arteries. These anomalous origins of the renal arteries are commonly seen in individuals with ectopic or horseshoe kidneys.

▷Rumwell CB, McPharlin M: *Vascular Technology: An Illustrated Review*, 5th edition. Pasadena, CA, Davies Publishing, 2015, p 8.

64.   B. Superior mesenteric.

The superior mesenteric artery (SMA) is the second major branch of the abdominal aorta. It arises approximately 1 cm below the origin of the celiac trunk. Major branches of the SMA include the inferior pancreaticoduodenal artery, jejunal and ileal branches, ileocolic artery, right colic artery, and the middle colic artery. The inferior mesenteric artery (IMA) feeds the left third of the transverse colon, the sigmoid colon, and part of the rectum. It is usually much smaller than the SMA. It arises on the left ventral aspect of the abdominal aorta a few centimeters before the aortic bifurcation. Its major branches include the left colic artery, sigmoid branches, and superior rectal artery.

▷Rumwell CB, McPharlin M: *Vascular Technology: An Illustrated Review*, 5th edition. Pasadena, CA, Davies Publishing, 2015, p 8.

65.   D. Internal iliac artery.

66.   A. Splenic artery.

67.   A. Arcuate arteries.

The main renal artery divides at the hilum of the kidney into segmental renal arteries. These in turn give rise to the interlobar arteries, which course alongside the renal pyramids. The arcuate arteries arise at right angles from the interlobar arteries and course on top of the renal pyramids. Within the renal cortex, the arcuate arteries give rise to the radially oriented interlobular arteries.

68.   C. Capillaries.

69.   B. The outer lining of the arterial wall.

▷Rumwell CB, McPharlin M: *Vascular Technology: An Illustrated Review*, 5th edition. Pasadena, CA, Davies Publishing, 2015, p 13.

▷Belanger A: *Vascular Anatomy and Physiology*. Pasadena, CA, Davies Publishing, 1999, p 24.

70.   A. The inner lining of the arterial wall.

▷Rumwell CB, McPharlin M: *Vascular Technology: An Illustrated Review*, 5th edition. Pasadena, CA, Davies Publishing, 2015, p 12.

▷Belanger A: *Vascular Anatomy and Physiology*. Pasadena, CA, Davies Publishing, 1999, p 24.

71.   B. Vasa vasorum.

Vasa vasorum is Latin for "vessel-vessels"—i.e., vasculature to perfuse the tissue of the vasculature.

▷Rumwell CB, McPharlin M: *Vascular Technology: An Illustrated Review*, 5th edition. Pasadena, CA, Davies Publishing, 2015, p 204.

▷Belanger A: *Vascular Anatomy and Physiology*. Pasadena, CA, Davies Publishing, 1999, p 25.

72. C. Tunica intima.

▷Belanger A: *Vascular Anatomy and Physiology*. Pasadena, CA, Davies Publishing, 1999, p 21–36.

73. A. This statement about capillaries—"They have only intima and adventitia layers"—is false.

Capillaries are made only of endothelial cells—just intima.

▷Rumwell CB, McPharlin M: *Vascular Technology: An Illustrated Review*, 5th edition. Pasadena, CA, Davies Publishing, 2015, p 12.

74. C. Tunica adventitia and tunica intima.

▷Belanger A: *Vascular Anatomy and Physiology*. Pasadena, CA, Davies Publishing, 1999, p 21–36.

CEREBROVASCULAR DISEASE

75. B. Intima.

The intimal lining of endothelial cells becomes disrupted in the first stage of the atherosclerotic process.

▷Pellerito JS, Polak JF: *Introduction to Vascular Ultrasonography*, 6th edition. Philadelphia, Elsevier Saunders, 2012, p 136.

76. B. Female gender.

Being female is not considered a risk factor, although postmenopausal females are at greater risk for atherosclerosis than premenopausal females. Indeed, male gender is considered a (minor) risk factor. Darn.

▷Hiatt WR, Cooke JP: Atherogenesis and the medical management of atherosclerosis. In Rutherford RB (ed): *Vascular Surgery*, 5th edition. Philadelphia, Saunders, 2000, p 334.

77. D. All of the above.

Ulceration of atherosclerotic plaque can be described as erosion of the intimal layer over the plaque surface. The erosion may progress to deep ulceration with embolization of plaque fragments. Thrombus formation is initiated by erosion of the plaque surface. Platelet aggregation occurs, forming a thrombus directly over the ulceration. Distal embolization of thrombus fragments may be the source of TIAs. Intraplaque hemorrhage can occur as leakage of blood into the atherosclerotic plaque through the ulceration or by rupture of the vaso vasorum.

▷Rumwell CB, McPharlin M: *Vascular Technology: An Illustrated Review*, 5th edition. Pasadena, CA, Davies Publishing, 2015, pp 210–213.

78. B. Females.

▷Stanley JC, Wakefield TW: Arterial fibrodysplasia. In Rutherford RB (ed): *Vascular Surgery*, 5th edition. Philadelphia, Saunders, 2000, p 401.

79. C. This statement—"Atherosclerosis is a red blood cell disease"—is NOT true.

Atherosclerosis is a generalized disease that begins most often at bifurcations due to the shear forces generated at the wall surfaces. Patients with atherosclerosis in the periphery will have other atherosclerotic changes in the carotid and coronary vessels even though these may be clinically silent. Disruption of intimal continuity is the primary initial manifestation.

▷Sidawy AN, Mitchell ME: Basic considerations of the arterial wall in health and disease. In Rutherford RB (ed): *Vascular Surgery*, 5th edition. Philadelphia, Saunders, 2000, p 60 ff.

80. E. Innominate artery occlusion.

If the innominate were involved, it would lower pressure on the right, not the left. The other answer choices are at least dimly possible, if not always likely.

81. E. None of the above will necessarily be present.

All of the answer choices are possible with right subclavian stenosis, but whether they actually occur depends on the severity of the stenosis.

82. G. A and B.

To produce a vertebral steal, the lesion must be proximal to the vertebral artery, creating an abnormal pressure gradient that pulls blood from the vertebral artery to perfuse the arm. Occlusion of the common carotid artery would not create this gradient, and the axillary artery is too far distal.

▷Rumwell CB, McPharlin M: *Vascular Technology: An Illustrated Review*, 5th edition. Pasadena, CA, Davies Publishing, 2015, pp 249–251.

83. C. Occlusion of the common carotid artery.

A bruit is the result of vibration in the tissue surrounding a stenotic vessel. An occluded vessel cannot produce a bruit.

84. C. Atherosclerosis.

▷Hiatt WR, Cooke JP: Atherogenesis and the medical management of atherosclerosis. In Rutherford RB (ed): *Vascular Surgery*, 5th edition. Philadelphia, Saunders, 2000, p 337.

85. A. Cardiac-source embolization.

Atrial fibrillation and myocardial infarction are the two most common causes of mural thrombus in the heart. Answer B is a remote possibility; it can happen.

▷Bernstein EF: The clinical spectrum of ischemic cerebrovascular disease. In Bernstein EF (ed): *Vascular Diagnosis*, 4th edition. St. Louis, Mosby, 1993, p 289.

86. C. Hypertension.

▷Rumwell CB, McPharlin M: *Vascular Technology: An Illustrated Review*, 5th edition. Pasadena, CA, Davies Publishing, 2015, p 210.

87. A. Origin of the internal carotid artery.

▷Rumwell CB, McPharlin M: *Vascular Technology: An Illustrated Review*, 5th edition. Pasadena, CA, Davies Publishing, 2015, p 211.

88. E. Ischemic.

Approximately 85% of strokes are ischemic in nature; only 15% of strokes are caused by intracerebral hemorrhage. Strokes caused by hemorrhage, however, account for most stroke fatalities.

▷Rumwell CB, McPharlin M: *Vascular Technology: An Illustrated Review*, 5th edition. Pasadena, CA, Davies Publishing, 2015, pp 210–211.

89. C. Between the internal and external carotid arteries.

▷Rumwell CB, McPharlin M: *Vascular Technology: An Illustrated Review*, 5th edition. Pasadena, CA, Davies Publishing, 2015, p 214.

90. C. This statement about subclavian steal—"It results from severe stenosis or occlusion of the proximal vertebral artery"—is NOT true.

All other statements are correct. In subclavian steal, a severe stenosis or occlusion is present in the proximal subclavian artery. This results in retrograde flow in the ipsilateral vertebral artery, as illustrated in the drawing below. The flow is "stolen" from the contralateral vertebral artery by way of the basilar artery.

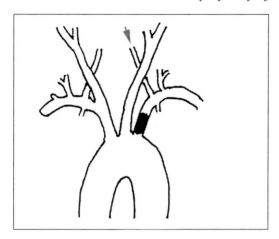

Although subclavian steals occur most frequently on the left side, they are seen on the right occasionally with obstruction of the proximal right subclavian or innominate artery. Most subclavian steals are asymptomatic. When symptoms do occur, the term <u>subclavian steal syndrome</u> is used to describe the condition. The symptoms associated with subclavian steal include dizziness, vertigo, diplopia, ataxia, and bilaterally blurred vision. Arm claudication or numbness is not common, but may occur in approximately one-third of patients.

▷Rumwell CB, McPharlin M: *Vascular Technology: An Illustrated Review*, 5th edition. Pasadena, CA, Davies Publishing, 2015, pp 249–250.

▷Ku DN, Lumsden A: Blood flow patterns in cerebrovascular disease. In Bernstein EF (ed): *Noninvasive Diagnostic Techniques in Vascular Disease*. St. Louis, Mosby, 1985, pp 73–83.

91. A. Carotid dissection.

Any kind of severe inertial injury, as with the sudden and violent movement of a car accident, can cause a tearing injury to the aorta or other arteries. A patient this young is unlikely to have atherosclerotic carotid disease. Cerebral aneurysm is more distantly possible, but the history of automobile accident makes carotid dissection the best answer.

▷Rumwell CB, McPharlin M: *Vascular Technology: An Illustrated Review*, 5th edition. Pasadena, CA, Davies Publishing, 2015, p 215.

92. E. Neointimal hyperplasia.

This is a common phenomenon following any trauma to an arterial wall, including endarterectomy and angioplasty. It involves proliferation of smooth-muscle cells in response to the injury.

▷Rumwell CB, McPharlin M: *Vascular Technology: An Illustrated Review*, 5th edition. Pasadena, CA, Davies Publishing, 2015, p 216.

▷Clowes AW: Pathologic intimal hyperplasia as a response to vascular injury and reconstruction. In Rutherford RB (ed): *Vascular Surgery*, 5th edition. Philadelphia, Saunders, 2000, p 409.

93.   B. Weakness of one side.

Hemiparesis is also referred to as unilateral paresis.

▷Rumwell CB, McPharlin M: *Vascular Technology: An Illustrated Review*, 5th edition. Pasadena, CA, Davies Publishing, 2015, p 217.

94.   D. Diameter percentage stenosis calculated by dividing the minimal diameter by the diameter of the unstenosed distal internal carotid artery.

Many studies prior to the NASCET study used the maximum diameter of the carotid bulb as the reference. Since an angiogram cannot accurately determine the outer diameter of the bulb, this method has probably caused inaccurate results. On the other hand, our diagnostic velocity criteria were based on the old method, which makes correlation with angiography more complex.

▷Pellerito JS, Polak JF: *Introduction to Vascular Ultrasonography*, 6th edition. Philadelphia, Elsevier Saunders, 2012, p 93.

95.   E. Amaurosis fugax.

Amaurosis fugax is transient blindness, usually in one eye. Lateralizing symptoms are usually from the anterior circulation, whereas nonlateralizing ischemic attacks, such as answers A, B, C, and D, are usually from the posterior circulation.

▷Rumwell CB, McPharlin M: *Vascular Technology: An Illustrated Review*, 5th edition. Pasadena, CA, Davies Publishing, 2015, p 218.

96.   False: Homonymous hemianopia.

▷Rumwell CB, McPharlin M: *Vascular Technology: An Illustrated Review*, 5th edition. Pasadena, CA, Davies Publishing, 2015, p 218.

97.   D. Diplopia.

Diplopia—double vision—is a symptom of vertebrobasilar insufficiency.

▷Rumwell CB, McPharlin M: *Vascular Technology: An Illustrated Review*, 5th edition. Pasadena, CA, Davies Publishing, 2015, p 219.

98.   True: This is a Hollenhorst plaque.

These patients have a 75% risk of TIA or stroke over the next several years.

▷Bernstein EF: The clinical spectrum of ischemic
cerebrovascular disease. In Bernstein EF (ed): *Vascular
Diagnosis*, 4th edition. St. Louis, Mosby, 1993, p 292.

No, you won't see questions in this format on the registry exam.

99.   D. Amaurosis fugax.

*By definition amaurosis fugax is a unilateral symptom that is temporary in nature. It is
frequently described by the patient as a curtain or a shade that blocks vision temporarily.*

▷Rumwell CB, McPharlin M: *Vascular Technology: An
Illustrated Review*, 5th edition. Pasadena, CA, Davies
Publishing, 2015, p 218.

100. C. 500,000.

▷Zwiebel WJ: *Introduction to Vascular Ultrasonography*, 5th
edition. Philadelphia, Elsevier Saunders, 2005, p 107.

101. C. Transient ischemic attack.

▷Rumwell CB, McPharlin M: *Vascular Technology: An
Illustrated Review*, 5th edition. Pasadena, CA, Davies
Publishing, 2015, p 209.

102. B. The left side of the body.

*Transient ischemic attacks affect the side of the body opposite that of the ischemic
hemisphere.*

▷Rumwell CB, McPharlin M: *Vascular Technology: An
Illustrated Review*, 5th edition. Pasadena, CA, Davies
Publishing, 2015, p 219.

103. B. Temporary blindness or shading of the ipsilateral eye.

*Amaurosis fugax affects the same side, since thromboembolic activity from ulcerated
ipsilateral carotid atheroma is suspected.*

▷Rumwell CB, McPharlin M: *Vascular Technology: An
Illustrated Review*, 5th edition. Pasadena, CA, Davies
Publishing, 2015, p 219.

104. A. Resolves within 24 hours.

*Transient ischemic attacks (TIAs), by definition, resolve within 24 hours, although TIAs
often last just a few minutes.*

▷Rumwell CB, McPharlin M: *Vascular Technology: An Illustrated Review*, 5th edition. Pasadena, CA, Davies Publishing, 2015, p 209.

105. A. The vertebrobasilar arteries.

Bilateral ocular symptoms usually originate in the posterior circulation, as the visual cortex is in the occipital lobe. However, the specific binocular symptom of homonymous hemianopia (see above) results from obstruction of a middle cerebral artery branch, not the vertebrobasilar system.

▷Rumwell CB, McPharlin M: *Vascular Technology: An Illustrated Review*, 5th edition. Pasadena, CA, Davies Publishing, 2015, p 218.

▷Bernstein EF: The clinical spectrum of ischemic cerebrovascular disease. In Bernstein EF (ed): *Vascular Diagnosis*, 4th edition. St. Louis, Mosby, 1993, p 291.

106. B. Vertigo.

Bilateral or global symptoms are more likely to be from the vertebrobasilar system.

▷Rumwell CB, McPharlin M: *Vascular Technology: An Illustrated Review*, 5th edition. Pasadena, CA, Davies Publishing, 2015, p 218.

107. E. Facial asymmetry.

Dizziness, ataxia, or other bilateral/global symptoms (such as bilateral concurrent vision loss) come from the vertebrobasilar system. Facial asymmetry (i.e., lateralizing weakness) is a carotid—territory symptom.

▷Rumwell CB, McPharlin M: *Vascular Technology: An Illustrated Review*, 5th edition. Pasadena, CA, Davies Publishing, 2015, p 219.

108. E. A neurologic ischemic deficit that resolves completely after 24 hours.

The term reversible ischemic neurologic deficit (RIND) describes an intracranial ischemic event that does not resolve within 24 hours but thereafter completely resolves. An unreversed deficit is a stroke, also called a cerebrovascular accident (CVA).

▷Rumwell CB, McPharlin M: *Vascular Technology: An Illustrated Review*, 5th edition. Pasadena, CA, Davies Publishing, 2015, p 209.

109. D. Stroke.

Because it has persisted longer than 24 hours and has not resolved completely, it is a stroke.

▷Bernstein EF: The clinical spectrum of ischemic cerebrovascular disease. In Bernstein EF (ed): *Vascular Diagnosis*, 4th edition. St. Louis, Mosby, 1993, p 289.

110. B. Transient ischemic attack.

Since amaurosis fugax is, by definition, transient, it can best be described as a transient ischemic attack of the eye. "Stroke of the eye" would not be accurate, as that would imply tissue necrosis and permanent damage.

▷Rumwell CB, McPharlin M: *Vascular Technology: An Illustrated Review*, 5th edition. Pasadena, CA, Davies Publishing, 2015, p 218.

111. E. Symptom associated with vertebrobasilar insufficiency.

Dysphagia (with a "g") is difficulty with swallowing.

▷Rumwell CB, McPharlin M: *Vascular Technology: An Illustrated Review*, 5th edition. Pasadena, CA, Davies Publishing, 2015, p 219.

112. D. Homonymous hemianopia.

▷Rumwell CB, McPharlin M: *Vascular Technology: An Illustrated Review*, 5th edition. Pasadena, CA, Davies Publishing, 2015, p 218.

113. E. Tingling sensation.

▷Rumwell CB, McPharlin M: *Vascular Technology: An Illustrated Review*, 5th edition. Pasadena, CA, Davies Publishing, 2015, p 217.

114. A. Dysphasia.

"Aphasia" is widely used as well, but technically this is incorrect, since it means "absence of speech."

▷Rumwell CB, McPharlin M: *Vascular Technology: An Illustrated Review*, 5th edition. Pasadena, CA, Davies Publishing, 2015, p 217.

115. B. Left hemisphere.

The speech area of the cortex is in the temporal lobe of the dominant hemisphere.

▷Rumwell CB, McPharlin M: *Vascular Technology: An Illustrated Review*, 5th edition. Pasadena, CA, Davies Publishing, 2015, p 217.

116. G. B and C.

Subclavian steal is generally a benign disorder. The abnormal flow pattern is caused by arterial obstruction proximal to the origin of the vertebral artery. This creates an

abnormal pressure gradient that pulls—or "steals"—flow from the vertebral artery to perfuse the ipsilateral upper extremity.

▷Rumwell CB, McPharlin M: *Vascular Technology: An Illustrated Review*, 5th edition. Pasadena, CA, Davies Publishing, 2015, pp 249–250.

▷Pellerito JS, Polak JF: *Introduction to Vascular Ultrasonography*, 6th edition. Philadelphia, Elsevier Saunders, 2012, pp 119–120, 216–217.

117. B. More often on the left side.

▷Rumwell CB, McPharlin M: *Vascular Technology: An Illustrated Review*, 5th edition. Pasadena, CA, Davies Publishing, 2015, p 249.

▷Carter SA: Clinical problems in peripheral arterial disease: is the clinical diagnosis adequate. In Bernstein EF (ed): *Vascular Diagnosis*, 4th edition. St. Louis, Mosby, 1993, p 477.

118. E. The middle cerebral artery distribution and the contralateral side of the body.

▷Rumwell CB, McPharlin M: *Vascular Technology: An Illustrated Review*, 5th edition. Pasadena, CA, Davies Publishing, 2015, p 217.

119. C. Internal carotid artery.

▷Bernstein EF: The clinical spectrum of ischemic cerebrovascular disease. In Bernstein EF (ed): *Vascular Diagnosis*, 4th edition. St. Louis, Mosby, 1993, p 288.

120. B. Common carotid stenosis if the contralateral pulse is normal.

Sometimes, however, the right neck pulse can feel reduced because of the larger muscles overlying the carotid.

▷Dilley RB: The history and physical examination in vascular disease. In Bernstein EF (ed): *Vascular Diagnosis*, 4th edition. St. Louis, Mosby, 1993, p 8.

121. B. This statement—"The absence of the bruit rules out significant stenosis"—is NOT true.

Bruits are caused by turbulent flow. Presence of a bruit is significant, since there is turbulent flow for some reason (not always stenosis). The absence of a bruit does not rule out stenosis; severe stenosis may not cause a bruit.

▷Rumwell CB, McPharlin M: *Vascular Technology: An Illustrated Review*, 5th edition. Pasadena, CA, Davies Publishing, 2015, pp 219–220.

▷Dilley RB: The history and physical examination in vascular disease. In Bernstein EF (ed): *Vascular Diagnosis*, 4th edition. St. Louis, Mosby, 1993, p 8.

▷Hodges TC: Natural history of carotid stenosis. In Bernstein EF (ed): *Vascular Diagnosis*, 4th edition. St. Louis, Mosby, 1993, p 417.

122. A. Aortic valve stenosis.

Aortic murmurs radiate distally, frequently into the low carotids.

▷Dilley RB: The history and physical examination in vascular
disease. In Bernstein EF (ed): *Vascular Diagnosis*, 4th edition.
St. Louis, Mosby, 1993, p 8.

123. E. Innominate occlusion.

Innominate occlusion would be expected to make the right carotid pulse weaker, not stronger.

124. F. B, C, and D.

▷Rumwell CB, McPharlin M: *Vascular Technology: An
Illustrated Review*, 5th edition. Pasadena, CA, Davies
Publishing, 2015, pp 219–220.

▷Dilley RB: The history and physical examination in vascular
disease. In Bernstein EF (ed): *Vascular Diagnosis*, 4th edition.
St. Louis, Mosby, 1993, p 8.

▷Hodges TC: Natural history of carotid disease. In Bernstein
EF (ed): *Vascular Diagnosis*, 4th edition. St. Louis, Mosby,
1993, p 417.

125. D. Highly significant.

*Bruits are not always a reliable indicator of disease, but a bruit that extends into diastole
is highly significant for carotid artery stenosis or for any other arterial location. (Perhaps
this is related to the fact that elevated end-diastolic velocities are suggestive of severe
stenosis.)*

▷Dilley RB: The history and physical examination in vascular
disease. In Bernstein EF (ed): *Vascular Diagnosis*, 4th edition.
St. Louis, Mosby, 1993, p 8.

126. E. Critical preocclusive stenosis of the internal carotid artery.

Bruits in the neck often disappear when the stenosis is very high-grade or preocclusive.

▷Rumwell CB, McPharlin M: *Vascular Technology: An
Illustrated Review*, 5th edition. Pasadena, CA, Davies
Publishing, 2015, pp 219–220.

▷Zwiebel WJ: *Introduction to Vascular Ultrasonography*, 5th
edition. Philadelphia, Elsevier Saunders, 2005, p 183, Table
9-3. Note falling off of velocities with very severe stenosis.

127. C. The brachial blood pressures are compared to see if they are equal.

*If one pressure is 15–20 mmHg less than the other, subclavian steal is suspected on the
side of the lower pressure.*

▷Rumwell CB, McPharlin M: *Vascular Technology: An Illustrated Review*, 5th edition. Pasadena, CA, Davies Publishing, 2015, pp 249–250.

128. C. This statement—"the beam is continuously transmitted with intermittent reception according to vessel depth"—is false.

With pulsed-wave Doppler, the signal is transmitted in short bursts (or pulses), and the transducer "listens" for the reflected signal in between the transmitted pulses.

129. A. Flow turbulence.

The spectral window is the blank area underneath systole on the spectral waveform. It is filled in or "lost" when turbulent flow creates spectral broadening. Other reasons for loss of the spectral window include overuse of Doppler gain and incorrect positioning of the sample volume outside of the center streamline (depicting signals from the vessel wall or adjacent slower moving blood flow).

130. D. Carotid body tumor.

▷Rumwell CB, McPharlin M: *Vascular Technology: An Illustrated Review*, 5th edition. Pasadena, CA, Davies Publishing, 2015, p 214.

▷Pellerito JS, Polak JF: *Introduction to Vascular Ultrasonography*, 6th edition. Philadelphia, Elsevier Saunders, 2012, pp 181–183.

131. A. 90°.

Since the angle of incidence equals the angle of reflectance, more echoes return to the transducer with a 90° angle.

▷Ridgway DP: *Introduction to Vascular Scanning*, 4th edition. Pasadena, CA, Davies Publishing, 2014, pp 144–145, 157.

132. D. Greatly increased mean velocities in the middle cerebral artery.

Vasospasm causes greatly increased mean velocities in cerebral arteries.

▷Pellerito JS, Polak JF: *Introduction to Vascular Ultrasonography*, 6th edition. Philadelphia, Elsevier Saunders, 2012, pp 217–219.

133. B. Away from the beam.

From the suboccipital (foramen magnum) approach, flow should normally be away from the beam.

▷Rumwell CB, McPharlin M: *Vascular Technology: An Illustrated Review*, 5th edition. Pasadena, CA, Davies Publishing, 2015, p 242.

▷Pellerito JS, Polak JF: *Introduction to Vascular Ultrasonography*, 6th edition. Philadelphia, Elsevier Saunders, 2012, p 205.

134. E. Temporal arteritis.

▷Pellerito JS, Polak JF: *Introduction to Vascular Ultrasonography*, 6th edition. Philadelphia, Elsevier Saunders, 2012, pp 202–225.

135. D. 60°.

It is generally accepted that, to make consistent velocity measurements, one must be consistent about the Doppler beam angle. Some labs insist on 60°, no more and no less; other labs keep it within the range of 45° or 50° to 60°.

▷Rumwell CB, McPharlin M: *Vascular Technology: An Illustrated Review*, 5th edition. Pasadena, CA, Davies Publishing, 2015, p 223.

136. B. 2 MHz.

▷Pellerito JS, Polak JF: *Introduction to Vascular Ultrasonography*, 6th edition. Philadelphia, Elsevier Saunders, 2012, p 202.

137. B. Away from the beam.

▷Pellerito JS, Polak JF: *Introduction to Vascular Ultrasonography*, 6th edition. Philadelphia, Elsevier Saunders, 2012, p 205.

138. E. Significant stenosis of the middle cerebral artery.

▷Pellerito JS, Polak JF: *Introduction to Vascular Ultrasonography*, 6th edition. Philadelphia, Elsevier Saunders, 2012, p 212.

139. A. 0°.

This appears to work fairly well, even though obviously some of the angles of incidence relative to flow are well away from 0°. (Note that, even with a 30° deviation of angle from 0°, the error in velocity estimate is only approximately 5%.)

▷Rumwell CB, McPharlin M: *Vascular Technology: An Illustrated Review*, 5th edition. Pasadena, CA, Davies Publishing, 2015, p 240.

140. A. Ipsilateral carotid obstruction, with right-to-left collateralization.

Flow in the ACA is normally away from the beam, so this is not normal. It suggests flow coming across from the other hemisphere via the anterior communicating artery.

▷Pellerito JS, Polak JF: *Introduction to Vascular Ultrasonography*, 6th edition. Philadelphia, Elsevier Saunders, 2012, p 218.

141. E. A and B.

Anatomic narrowing of an artery can increase the velocity; increasing the operating or transmitted frequency will increase the frequency shift (see the Doppler equation). Readjusting the angle-correct cursor will change the velocity estimate for a given frequency shift, but won't change the shift itself. The threshold sensitivity does not affect frequency shift.

142. E. Elevation of systolic frequency with poststenotic turbulence.

The most sensitive parameter for calling this degree of stenosis is the systolic frequency/velocity. Focal acceleration with distal turbulence is the hallmark of significant stenosis anywhere in the body.

▷Rumwell CB, McPharlin M: *Vascular Technology: An Illustrated Review*, 5th edition. Pasadena, CA, Davies Publishing, 2015, pp 234–235.

143. D. Place transducer and acoustic gel within a sterile sleeve or bag.

Autoclaving a transducer will destroy its piezoelectric properties.

144. E. Increasing the beam angle to 70°.

This would create a lower frequency shift than the proper 60° angle (Doppler equation again). The other choices would more likely increase, not decrease, the frequency shift.

▷Pellerito JS, Polak JF: *Introduction to Vascular Ultrasonography*, 6th edition. Philadelphia, Elsevier Saunders, 2012, pp 244–247.

145. B. This statement about CW Doppler—"It allows more precise range-gating than pulse-wave Doppler"—is false.

Continuous-wave Doppler cannot range-gate; information is returned from along the entire beam.

▷Pellerito JS, Polak JF: *Introduction to Vascular Ultrasonography*, 6th edition. Philadelphia, Elsevier Saunders, 2012, pp 38–39.

146. A. Depth information is not possible; precise location of flow pattern cannot be determined.

The two-transducer probes for continuous-wave (CW) Doppler are relatively inexpensive. Directionality is included in most diagnostic-grade CW Doppler systems, and they can be connected to a spectrum analyzer. And of course CW has no sample volume as pulsed Doppler does. (See above.)

▷Pellerito JS, Polak JF: *Introduction to Vascular Ultrasonography*, 6th edition. Philadelphia, Elsevier Saunders, 2012, pp 38–39.

147. A. This spectrum is characteristic of an external carotid artery.

This waveform has a prominent dicrotic notch, a sharp peak, and relatively little diastolic flow. We don't know for sure that it is the ECA, but it is characteristic of that artery. The common carotid artery might have similar-appearing peaks, but normally it would have more diastolic flow.

▷Pellerito JS, Polak JF: *Introduction to Vascular Ultrasonography*, 6th edition. Philadelphia, Elsevier Saunders, 2012, p 139.

148. C. This spectrum is characteristic of an internal carotid artery.

This waveform has lots of diastolic flow, a less distinct peak, and a less prominent dicrotic notch. It is characteristic of the ICA or of any artery feeding a low-resistance distal bed, such as a renal artery.

▷Pellerito JS, Polak JF: *Introduction to Vascular Ultrasonography*, 6th edition. Philadelphia, Elsevier Saunders, 2012, p 139.

149. E. This statement—"The velocities suggest severe (greater than 80%) stenosis"—is false.

This waveform has a significantly elevated peak systolic velocity (>125 cm/sec), and the systolic window is filled in, suggesting fairly severe turbulence. However, the end-diastolic velocities are not greatly elevated, certainly not approaching 100 cm/sec. Therefore, based on this information, this stenosis would be called hemodynamically significant but not severe (i.e., > 50%, not > 80%).

▷Rumwell CB, McPharlin M: *Vascular Technology: An Illustrated Review*, 5th edition. Pasadena, CA, Davies Publishing, 2015, pp 234–235.

150. C. The elevated peak-systolic velocities and significant end-diastolic velocities suggest significant ICA stenosis (> 50% by diameter).

The PSV of 285 cm/sec is decidedly high enough to call >50%, well over the time-honored and still valid criterion of >125 cm/sec for this threshold. On the other hand, nearly all criteria would call for higher PSV and especially higher EDV to call >80%. The systolic window is not filled: flow is still reasonably orderly here, but the elevated velocities do suggest hemodynamically-significant stenosis.

▷Rumwell CB, McPharlin M: *Vascular Technology: An Illustrated Review*, 5th edition. Pasadena, CA, Davies Publishing, 2015, pp 234–235.

151. A. Toward the beam.

▷Rumwell CB, McPharlin M: *Vascular Technology: An Illustrated Review*, 5th edition. Pasadena, CA, Davies Publishing, 2015, p 242.

152. E. A, B, and C.

Beam width relates to lateral resolution.

▷Pellerito JS, Polak JF: *Introduction to Vascular Ultrasonography*, 6th edition. Philadelphia, Elsevier Saunders, 2012, pp 26–29.

153. E. A and B.

Both 5 MHz and 10 MHz transducers can be used to scan the carotids.

▷Rumwell CB, McPharlin M: *Vascular Technology: An Illustrated Review*, 5th edition. Pasadena, CA, Davies Publishing, 2015, p 224.

154. F. B and C.

▷Pellerito JS, Polak JF: *Introduction to Vascular Ultrasonography*, 6th edition. Philadelphia, Elsevier Saunders, 2012, pp 30–31.

155. C. Middle cerebral artery.

▷Rumwell CB, McPharlin M: *Vascular Technology: An Illustrated Review*, 5th edition. Pasadena, CA, Davies Publishing, 2015, p 242.

156. B. As small as possible, to resolve side-by-side lesions

Again, we're having some occasional overlap with physics matters.

▷Pellerito JS, Polak JF: *Introduction to Vascular Ultrasonography*, 6th edition. Philadelphia, Elsevier Saunders, 2012, pp 30–31.

157. A. Temporal.

▷Rumwell CB, McPharlin M: *Vascular Technology: An Illustrated Review*, 5th edition. Pasadena, CA, Davies Publishing, 2015, p 240.

158. A. A mosaic of low red and blue frequencies in color flow in tissue lying outside of the lumen, and oscillatory waveforms above and below baseline in the spectral waveform.

The frequencies associated with a bruit are low rather than high. Low-frequency oscillations above and below a spectral baseline that are characteristic of a bruit may also show as low-frequency red and blue color shifts in adjacent tissue, often speckled like a mosaic.

▷Rutherford RB (ed): *Vascular Surgery*, 5th edition.
Philadelphia, Saunders, 2000, Plate VII at the beginning of the
book for a good illustration of both phenomena.

159. C. Retrograde flow in the distal internal carotid artery.

While the flow in the segment of the carotid artery distal to a new total occlusion conceivably could have eddy currents, it could not have purely retrograde flow. An important fact to remember is that, with rare exceptions, occluded internal carotid arteries may not be reconstructed by surgical means.

▷Rumwell CB, McPharlin M: *Vascular Technology: An
Illustrated Review*, 5th edition. Pasadena, CA, Davies
Publishing, 2015, pp 228, 235.

160. A. Calcified plaque.

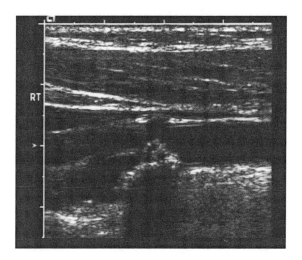

▷Pellerito JS, Polak JF: *Introduction to Vascular
Ultrasonography*, 6th edition. Philadelphia, Elsevier Saunders,
2012, pp 149–151.

161. D. Homogeneous plaque.

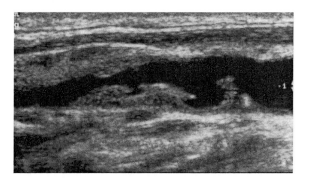

These echoes are soft and gray and have essentially the same character throughout (hence the term <u>homogeneous</u>). This plaque also has some rather forbidding-looking scooped-out areas, although of course duplex ultrasound does not have a strong track record in the literature for calling ulceration.

▷Pellerito JS, Polak JF: *Introduction to Vascular Ultrasonography*, 6th edition. Philadelphia, Elsevier Saunders, 2012, p 151.

▷Rumwell CB, McPharlin M: *Vascular Technology: An Illustrated Review*, 5th edition. Pasadena, CA, Davies Publishing, 2015, p 227.

162. C. Orbital.

▷Rumwell CB, McPharlin M: *Vascular Technology: An Illustrated Review*, 5th edition. Pasadena, CA, Davies Publishing, 2015, pp 240–241.

163. C. End-diastolic velocity.

This is the most widely used criterion, although of course no number all by itself should determine an interpretation. Some investigators have had success with velocity ratios (e.g., ICA/CCA systolic and/or diastolic ratios).

▷Rumwell CB, McPharlin M: *Vascular Technology: An Illustrated Review*, 5th edition. Pasadena, CA, Davies Publishing, 2015, pp 234–235.

164. D. 50%.

You can do the math if you like: A = πr^2 (diameter = 2 r). Use a 10 mm artery. Diameter reduction of 10 mm to 5 mm:

(10 – 5) ÷ 10 = 50%

Area reduction of (5 x 5) x 3.14 = 78.5 mm²
to
(2.5 x 2.5) x 3.14 = 19.6 mm²

(75 – 19.6) ÷ 75 = 74%

Okay, it's 74%, not 75%. Which one is easier to remember?

▷Rumwell CB, McPharlin M: *Vascular Technology: An Illustrated Review*, 5th edition. Pasadena, CA, Davies Publishing, 2015, pp 255–256.

165. A. 96%.

This dramatizes the very severe loss of cross-sectional area available for flow in a severe stenosis. (And for those who like to call "99% stenosis," that translates to a cross-sectional area of about, oh, let's see, 0.03 mm², or about 30 square microns. In other words, it gets to be a figure of speech more than an accurate estimate.) Casual use of both types of measurement can lead to serious misunderstanding (i.e., apples and oranges). In

this question, the true severity of the 80% diameter stenosis is emphasized by the loss of 96% of the lumen area—pretty dramatic. On the following page, there is a table to show the relationship at all levels:

% Diameter stenosis	% Corresponding area reduction
10	19
20	36
30	51
40	64
50	75
60	84
70	91
80	96
90	99

166. E. Color flow PRF set too low, creating aliasing and overestimation of velocities.

Apart from the fact that the color flow shouldn't be the only determining factor in interpreting the duplex study, this situation would be expected to overestimate stenosis, not to underestimate it.

The other scenarios are quite possible: A long, smooth stenosis will cause changes in flow character that are less pronounced than those caused by an abrupt and/or irregular stenosis. Assessing with just one longitudinal plane is a bad idea in both angiography and duplex ultrasonography. Sloppy angle correction can cause poor velocity estimates. And in the case of pronounced shadowing, you might need to assess on the basis of poststenotic turbulence as much as acceleration of flow.

▷Pellerito JS, Polak JF: *Introduction to Vascular Ultrasonography*, 6th edition. Philadelphia, Elsevier Saunders, 2012, p 148.

▷Rumwell CB, McPharlin M: *Vascular Technology: An Illustrated Review*, 5th edition. Pasadena, CA, Davies Publishing, 2015, p 256.

167. E. Basilar artery.

▷Rumwell CB, McPharlin M: *Vascular Technology: An Illustrated Review*, 5th edition. Pasadena, CA, Davies Publishing, 2015, pp 240–241.

168. B. High-resistance character in the ECA, low-resistance in the ICA, with mixed character in the CCA.

▷Pellerito JS, Polak JF: *Introduction to Vascular Ultrasonography*, 6th edition. Philadelphia, Elsevier Saunders, 2012, pp 140–141.

169. A. Small, to sample flow only from center stream.

170. A. Adjusted parallel with arterial walls.

> ▷Ridgway DP: *Introduction to Vascular Scanning*, 4th edition.
> Pasadena, CA, Davies Publishing, 2014, p 159.

171. D. Depth on the y-axis.

> ▷Ridgway DP: *Introduction to Vascular Scanning*, 4th edition.
> Pasadena, CA, Davies Publishing, 2014, p 79.

172. B.

This position creates angles too close to 90° to create a good color display.

> ▷Ridgway DP: *Introduction to Vascular Scanning*, 4th edition.
> Pasadena, CA, Davies Publishing, 2014, pp 362–364.

173. B. The frequency shifts are changing at different points in the color box due to the curvature of the artery.

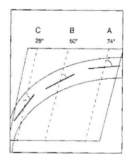

One must be constantly on the alert for changing angles, which create potentially misleading color flow changes.

> ▷Ridgway DP: *Introduction to Vascular Scanning*, 4th edition.
> Pasadena, CA, Davies Publishing, 2014, pp 367–368.

174. B. External carotid artery.

This percussion maneuver—the "temporal tap"— must be used only cautiously to help identify the ECA in difficult situations. One report suggests that you can get pretty good oscillations in the ICA with temporal artery percussions in a large proportion of patients. It is better to differentiate the ICA and ECA by evaluating waveform characteristics, vessel positions, and the presence of branches.

> ▷Pellerito JS, Polak JF: *Introduction to Vascular Ultrasonography*, 6th edition. Philadelphia, Elsevier Saunders, 2012, pp 140–141.

175. B. Increase color flow PRF.

Increasing PRF will make the color flow less sensitive to slow flow.

▷Pellerito JS, Polak JF: *Introduction to Vascular Ultrasonography*, 6th edition. Philadelphia, Elsevier Saunders, 2012, pp 174–176.

176. D. Greatly increased end-diastolic velocities in CCA spectral display.

The high distal resistance created by the ICA occlusion would reduce or eliminate diastolic flow in the CCA, not increase it.

▷Pellerito JS, Polak JF: *Introduction to Vascular Ultrasonography*, 6th edition. Philadelphia, Elsevier Saunders, 2012, pp 175–176.

177. C. Suggestive of developing subclavian steal syndrome.

The developing abnormal pressure gradient in the left arm is pulling flow below baseline at systole; the flow reverts to antegrade in diastole (referred to as a "to and fro" pattern in Zwiebel). This might be converted to a full steal by performing reactive hyperemia on the left arm or having the patient exercise the arm to increase demand.

▷Pellerito JS, Polak JF: *Introduction to Vascular Ultrasonography*, 6th edition. Philadelphia, Elsevier Saunders, 2012, p 197.

178. D. You should ask the patient to perform a Valsalva maneuver.

Vertebral venous signals can be quite convincingly pulsatile. It may help to swing up for a common carotid signal to establish which direction is antegrade if you aren't sure from the display.

179. B. The medial part of the frontal bone.

▷Pellerito JS, Polak JF: *Introduction to Vascular Ultrasonography*, 6th edition. Philadelphia, Elsevier Saunders, 2012, pp 204–205.

180. B. Genicular to arcuate branches.

Genicular arteries are around the knee; arcuate arteries are in the kidneys.

▷Pellerito JS, Polak JF: *Introduction to Vascular Ultrasonography*, 6th edition. Philadelphia, Elsevier Saunders, 2012, pp 111–113, 174–176.

181. B. The external carotid has branches near the bifurcation and the internal carotid does not.

▷Rumwell CB, McPharlin M: *Vascular Technology: An Illustrated Review*, 5th edition. Pasadena, CA, Davies Publishing, 2015, p 200.

182. B. Even double projection arteriography may fail to fully determine diameter stenosis, especially in the event of vessel overlap.

One of the main advantages of duplex is the ability to visualize in cross section to the artery. Vessel overlap is a common problem. A kink would show up on angiography. "Background ultrasound noise" would not cause accelerated velocities.

183. C. Inadvertent venous puncture.

Inadvertent venous puncture would not constitute a major complication; the others are much more severe outcomes.

▷Johnston KW: Overview. In Rutherford RB (ed): *Vascular Surgery*, 5th edition. Philadelphia, Saunders, 2000, p 625.

184. B. 1% of patients.

▷Bernstein EF: The clinical spectrum of ischemic cerebrovascular disease. In Bernstein EF (ed): *Vascular Diagnosis*, 4th edition. St. Louis, Mosby, 1993, p 293.

185. C. Degree of narrowing of ICA by cross-sectional area.

Angiograms are longitudinal pictures of vessels; they cannot provide cross-sectional information.

186. D. It is often nondiagnostic.

Despite some pitfalls, noted elsewhere, angiography is the definitive imaging study of the arterial system.

▷Bernstein EF: The clinical spectrum of ischemic cerebrovascular disease. In Bernstein EF (ed): *Vascular Diagnosis*, 4th edition. St. Louis, Mosby, 1993, p 293.

187. A. Common femoral artery.

▷Rumwell CB, McPharlin M: *Vascular Technology: An Illustrated Review*, 5th edition. Pasadena, CA, Davies Publishing, 2015, p 174.

188. D. Unlimited repeatability.

This is an invasive procedure with a small but definite risk of complication.

▷Zierler RE: Basic and practical aspects of cerebrovascular testing. In Bernstein EF (ed): *Vascular Diagnosis*, 4th edition. St. Louis, Mosby, 1993, p 308.

189. B. CT.

Computed tomography is the usual first choice of exam, since it can distinguish hemorrhagic stroke from ischemic infarction and is usually more readily available. In

addition, it is better tolerated because examination time is shorter. The other exams are quite possible as well, but less likely for initial evaluation.

▷Moore WD: Diagnosis, evaluation, and medical management of patients with ischemic cerebrovascular disease. In Rutherford RB (ed): *Vascular Surgery*, 5th edition. Philadelphia, Saunders, 2000, p 1736.

190. E. Radiofrequency pulses created by tissue and blood flow.

Magnetic resonance works by sending pulses of radio waves into tissue within a strong magnetic field. The resulting change of spin of the hydrogen protons create a signal that is then processed for image. Different processing methods ("time-of-flight" technique) can create images of blood flow; hence MR angiography or MRA.

▷Ricci MA, Knight SJ: The role of noninvasive studies in the diagnosis and management of cerebrovascular disease. In Rutherford RB (ed): *Vascular Surgery*, 5th edition. Philadelphia, Saunders, 2000, p 1785.

191. F. All but B.

MRA has become an accurate method for assessing carotid stenosis. Patients with pacemakers or other significant bodily metal cannot be subjected to the strong magnetic field this test requires. MRA uses radio waves, not ionizing radiation (e.g., x-rays). It does require the patient to lie quite still for a good while. It does tend to overestimate stenosis, while at least one study demonstrated that angiography often underestimates stenosis. Of course, we duplex users are always right on the money. (Once again, the ARDMS exam is unlikely to give you nine answers to choose from.)

▷Ricci MA, Knight SJ: The role of noninvasive studies in the diagnosis and management of cerebrovascular disease. In Rutherford RB (ed): *Vascular Surgery*, 5th edition. Philadelphia, Saunders, 2000, p 1785.

192. B. May be used for obstructed lower extremity arteries.

While endarterectomy is most often performed on carotid arteries and has been largely superceded in the lower extremity arteries by the use of bypass grafts, it is still sometimes a useful option for revascularization of iliac or femoral arteries. New techniques have improved the outcomes for this procedure in the lower extremity arteries.

▷Messina LM, Stoney RJ: Endarterectomy. In Rutherford RB (ed): *Vascular Surgery*, 5th edition. Philadelphia, Saunders, 2000, pp 493 ff.

193. B. Are technically less demanding than stenting of coronary arteries.

Stents (those little wire gizmos for holding arteries open) are now widely used in coronary and peripheral arteries, but their use in carotid arteries is controversial at this time. No long-term studies have demonstrated the safety or efficacy of this procedure, and it is not

significantly less expensive than surgery. It is indeed simpler from a purely technical standpoint to place a stent in a carotid artery than in coronary or peripheral arteries.

▷Deutsch LS: Anatomy and angiographic diagnosis of extracranial and intracranial vascular disease. In Rutherford RB (ed): *Vascular Surgery*, 5th edition. Philadelphia, Saunders, 2000, pp 1771–1773.

194. A. Carotid endarterectomy is probably recommended.

The symptomatology of a patient with any stenosis of the internal carotid artery makes it likely that endarterectomy will be recommended. Treatment of hypertension is usually a good idea, but is not the primary urgent issue here.

▷Pellerito JS, Polak JF: *Introduction to Vascular Ultrasonography*, 6th edition. Philadelphia, Elsevier Saunders, 2012, p 92.

195. C. Carotid endarterectomy for stenosis greater than 70% in diameter.

Carotid surgery is recommended for symptomatic patients in this trial.

▷Pellerito JS, Polak JF: *Introduction to Vascular Ultrasonography*, 6th edition. Philadelphia, Elsevier Saunders, 2012, p 92.

196. D. rtPA.

Recombinant tissue plasminogen activator (rtPA) is useful in improving outcomes only if administered within three hours of the onset of symptoms.

▷Hughes RL, Anderson CA, Sung GY: Diagnosis, evaluation, and medical management of patients with ischemic cerebrovascular disease. In Rutherford RB (ed): *Vascular Surgery*, 5th edition. Philadelphia, Saunders, 2000, p 1739.

197. D. After carotid endarterectomy.

Hyperperfusion after carotid endarterectomy is a potentially serious complication, one of the most common following carotid endarterectomy.

▷Sundt TM: Cerebral blood flow measurements during carotid endarterectomy. In Bernstein EF (ed): *Vascular Diagnosis*, 4th edition. St. Louis, Mosby, 1993, p 395.

VENOUS DISEASE

198. C. A 75-year-old woman admitted for transient ischemic attack.

Venous disease is not particularly prevalent in individuals admitted for carotid artery disease, though age is a risk factor. However, individuals with cancer, fractured hips, multiple injuries, CHF, and obesity are at greater risk for deep venous thrombosis.

▷Rumwell CB, McPharlin M: *Vascular Technology: An Illustrated Review*, 5th edition. Pasadena, CA, Davies Publishing, 2015, pp 283–284.

199. B. Pulmonary embolism may occur.

While damage to deep venous valves and pain are concerns with patients exhibiting acute deep venous thrombosis, the most severe manifestation and the biggest fear is that of pulmonary embolism. Pulmonary embolism is an extremely severe sequela of deep venous thrombosis.

▷Zwolak RM: Arterial duplex scanning. In Rutherford RB (ed): *Vascular Surgery*, 5th edition. Philadelphia, Saunders, 2000, p 208.

200. E. All except D.

▷Rumwell CB, McPharlin M: *Vascular Technology: An Illustrated Review*, 5th edition. Pasadena, CA, Davies Publishing, 2015, pp 285–286.

201. B. During muscle contraction.

Muscle contraction forces blood out to the superficial veins via incompetent perforating veins.

▷Zwolak RM: Arterial duplex scanning. In Rutherford RB (ed): *Vascular Surgery*, 5th edition. Philadelphia, Saunders, 2000, p 208.

202. A. Diabetes.

Diabetes is a risk factor for atherosclerosis, not deep venous thrombosis. All the rest are risk factors for DVT.

▷Rumwell CB, McPharlin M: *Vascular Technology: An Illustrated Review*, 5th edition. Pasadena, CA, Davies Publishing, 2015, pp 285–286.

203. E. Stasis, hypercoagulability, and intimal injury.

For DVT to occur, one or more of these conditions must be present. Virchow's triad: (1) Intimal injury, (2) hypercoagulability, and (3) stasis. The other answers refer either to later thrombotic stages or to atherosclerosis.

▷Rumwell CB, McPharlin M: *Vascular Technology: An Illustrated Review*, 5th edition. Pasadena, CA, Davies Publishing, 2015, pp 285–286.

204. D. Smoking.

Smoking is not one of the direct risk factors for DVT, although it is implicated when combined with birth control pills.

▷Rumwell CB, McPharlin M: *Vascular Technology: An Illustrated Review*, 5th edition. Pasadena, CA, Davies Publishing, 2015, p 286.

205. A. > 90%.

This explains the profound interest in diagnosing and treating deep venous thrombosis before it creates bigger problems.

▷Meissner MH, Strandness Jr DE: Pathophysiology and natural history of acute deep venous thrombosis. In Rutherford RB (ed): *Vascular Surgery*, 5th edition. Philadelphia, Saunders, 2000, p 1930.

206. A. Chronic but controllable.

Although it should be noted that some surgeons are replacing venous valves to "cure" venous incompetency, this is not yet standard treatment. It is difficult but possible to control the symptoms.

▷Moneta GL, Porter JM: Nonoperative treatment of chronic venous insufficiency. In Rutherford RB (ed): *Vascular Surgery*, 5th edition. Philadelphia, Saunders, 2000, p 1999.

207. A. Obesity.

Lymphatic dysfunction may be caused by any of the other causes B through E.

▷Gloviczki P, Wahner HW: Clinical diagnosis and evaluation of lymphedema. In Rutherford RB (ed): *Vascular Surgery*, 5th edition. Philadelphia, Saunders, 2000, p 2125 ff.

208. E. A dilatation of the great saphenous vein or superficial tributary.

Varicose veins usually affect the greater saphenous system and branches, whether they are primary or secondary varicosities.

▷Bergan JJ: Varicose veins: treatment by surgery and sclerotherapy. In Rutherford RB (ed): *Vascular Surgery*, 5th edition. Philadelphia, Saunders, 2000, p 2011.

209. B. Secondary varices.

As noted above, secondary varices result from chronic excessive intravenous pressure transmitted from the incompetent deep system.

▷Bergan JJ: Varicose veins: treatment by surgery and sclerotherapy. In Rutherford RB (ed): *Vascular Surgery*, 5th edition. Philadelphia, Saunders, 2000, p 2009.

210. A. Synovial fluid from the knee joint.

▷Zwiebel WJ: *Introduction to Vascular Ultrasonography*, 5th edition. Philadelphia, Elsevier Saunders, 2005, p 508.

211. D. The popliteal vein.

The gastroc veins empty into the popliteal vein. The soleal veins empty into the posterior tibial and peroneal veins.

▷Pellerito JS, Polak JF: *Introduction to Vascular Ultrasonography*, 6th edition. Philadelphia, Elsevier Saunders, 2012, p 368.

212. A. The posterior tibial veins.

Soleal veins drain into the posterior tibial and peroneal veins. It is thought that this is where much if not most of deep vein thrombosis begins.

▷Pellerito JS, Polak JF: *Introduction to Vascular Ultrasonography*, 6th edition. Philadelphia, Elsevier Saunders, 2012, p 367.

213. B. 15–20%.

Zwiebel says up to 28% and Pellerito says up to 30%. New information suggests two interesting things: (1) Perhaps about half of DVT does not involve the calf. (2) Many patients with isolated calf-vein thrombosis go on to have significant problems with chronic venous insufficiency and pulmonary embolism. (See Yearbook of Vascular Surgery 1999.)

▷Zwiebel WJ: *Introduction to Vascular Ultrasonography*, 5th edition. Philadelphia, Elsevier Saunders, 2005, pp 462–463.

▷Pellerito JS, Polak JF: *Introduction to Vascular Ultrasonography*, 6th edition. Philadelphia, Elsevier Saunders, 2012, p 345.

214. A. Damage to venous valves, allowing reflux.

▷Pellerito JS, Polak JF: *Introduction to Vascular Ultrasonography*, 6th edition. Philadelphia, Elsevier Saunders, 2012, pp 384–386.

215. D. Two of the above.

The obvious tentative call is deep vein thrombosis; a remoter possibility is traumatic AV fistula, which tends to increase distal venous pressure. Popliteal entrapment is not a likely call.

▷Sumner DS: Hemodynamics and pathophysiology of arteriovenous fistulae. In Rutherford RB (ed): *Vascular Surgery*, 5th edition. Philadelphia, Saunders, 2000, p 1404.

216. E. Gastrocnemius muscular thrombosis.

Isolated gastocnemius thrombosis is unlikely to create significant chronic venous insufficiency (CVI) symptoms. It is only fairly recently that we have come to know that even lesser saphenous insufficiency can cause stasis ulcers.

▷Moneta GL, Nehler MR, Porter JM: Pathophysiology of chronic venous insufficiency. In Rutherford RB (ed): *Vascular Surgery*, 5th edition. Philadelphia, Saunders, 2000, p 1985.

217. C. Relieved by elevation.

Elevation of the extremities decreases venous hypertension and pain.

▷Rutherford RB: Initial patient evaluation: the vascular consultation. In Rutherford RB (ed): *Vascular Surgery*, 5th edition. Philadelphia, Saunders, 2000, p 6.

218. B. 46–62% accurate.

The clinical diagnosis of deep venous thrombosis is only about 50% accurate, according to most studies. That means that there are a significant number of patients who, while they never have symptoms of deep venous thrombosis, nonetheless experience the disease. In addition, 50% of the people with all of the symptomatology of DVT do not have deep venous thrombosis. (Recent studies suggest that this dismal accuracy figure can be improved by narrowing the focus on symptoms to acute unilateral edema. However, this is a possible registry exam question for the time being.)

▷Rumwell CB, McPharlin M: *Vascular Technology: An Illustrated Review*, 5th edition. Pasadena, CA, Davies Publishing, 2015, p 283.

219. D. Swelling in the ankles and legs but not the feet.

Usually swelling is not found in the feet in venous disease.

▷Rutherford RB: Initial patient evaluation: the vascular consultation. In Rutherford RB (ed): *Vascular Surgery*, 5th edition. Philadelphia, Saunders, 2000, p 6.

220. D. Arthritis.

Of the answer choices, arthritis is the least likely cause of deep venous thrombosis. Patients with cancer are at increased risk because of systemic fibrinolytic changes.

▷Rumwell CB, McPharlin M: *Vascular Technology: An Illustrated Review*, 5th edition. Pasadena, CA, Davies Publishing, 2015, p 286.

221. C. Postphlebitic syndrome.

▷Rutherford RB: Initial patient evaluation: the vascular consultation. In Rutherford RB (ed): *Vascular Surgery*, 5th edition. Philadelphia, Saunders, 2000, p 6.

222. A. Recurrence of acute deep venous thrombosis.

Since previous DVT is a risk factor for new DVT, a sudden onset of new symptoms must be taken seriously.

▷Rumwell CB, McPharlin M: *Vascular Technology: An Illustrated Review*, 5th edition. Pasadena, CA, Davies Publishing, 2015, p 283 ff.

223. A. Cardiac or systemic origin.

Bilateral edema most commonly is cardiac or systemic in origin with congestive heart failure as a predominant feature.

▷Rutherford RB: Initial patient evaluation: the vascular consultation. In Rutherford RB (ed): *Vascular Surgery*, 5th edition. Philadelphia, Saunders, 2000, p 6.

224. F. B, C, and D.

Insufficiency may allow abnormal distal flow in the standing patient. If the patient is supine, hydrostatic pressure is not an issue, so venous pressure at the ankle would not be different from the non-insufficient patient. Walking creates hydrostatic increased pressure as a result of valvular insufficiency, along with a circular venous flow pattern that tends to keep more blood in the leg veins rather than moving it cephalad to the heart.

▷Sumner DS: Essential hemodynamic principles. In Rutherford RB (ed): *Vascular Surgery*, 5th edition. Philadelphia, Saunders, 2000, p 106.

225. B. They usually have a quick decrease in venous pressure that takes a minute or two to return to pre-exercise levels.

A prolonged return to pre-exercise pressure would be the normal response; return to maximum pressure should take a fairly long time in the patient with competent valves preventing reflux. In patients with incomplete recanalization of thrombus, the obstruction may even cause increased pressure with exercise because of congestion. Secondary varices may fill via incompetent perforators during exercise.

▷Sumner DS: Essential hemodynamic principles. In Rutherford RB (ed): *Vascular Surgery*, 5th edition. Philadelphia, Saunders, 2000, p 108.

226. B. Lymphedema.

Filaria is a nematode that takes up residence in the lymph system and can cause lymphedema. This would be a somewhat obscure differential diagnosis for deep venous thrombosis.

▷Gloviczki P, Wahner HW: Clinical diagnosis and evaluation of lymphedema. In Rutherford RB (ed): *Vascular Surgery*, 5th edition. Philadelphia, Saunders, 2000, p 2126.

227. A. IVC.

To create bilateral edema, thrombus would have to involve either both iliac veins or, more likely, the inferior vena cava. This situation might also cause renal dysfunction due to obstructed renal vein outflow.

▷Liddell RP, Dake MD: Endovascular treatment of chronic occlusions of large veins. In Rutherford RB (ed): *Vascular Surgery*, 5th edition. Philadelphia, Saunders, 2000, p 2073.

228. B. Venous disease.

You knew the answer, because this question isn't in the arterial section. In one survey, three-quarters of lower extremity ulcers were caused by chronic venous insufficiency.

▷Moneta GL, Nehler MR, Porter JM: Pathophysiology of chronic venous insufficiency. In Rutherford RB (ed): *Vascular Surgery*, 5th edition. Philadelphia, Saunders, 2000, p 1982.

229. D. Deep venous obstruction is present.

When deep venous obstruction is present, congestion and resulting increased deep venous pressure may back out into the perforating veins. With distension, valve leaflets cannot coapt, and flow can travel abnormally from deep to superficial veins. Secondary varicosities may result.

▷Pellerito JS, Polak JF: *Introduction to Vascular Ultrasonography*, 6th edition. Philadelphia, Elsevier Saunders, 2012, pp 383–384.

230. C. Cellulitis.

Cellulitis—inflammation of skin and deeper tissues caused by an infectious process—is one of the common differential diagnoses for deep venous thrombosis.

▷Oliver MA: Clinical evaluation. In Talbot SR, Oliver MA: *Techniques of Venous Imaging*. Pasadena, CA, Davies Publishing, 1992, p 32.

231. E. Rest pain.

Rest pain is a chronic arterial symptom. The others are symptoms of pulmonary embolism, many of which are quite similar to symptoms of myocardial infarction. [I had to go to an

old copy of Fahey's Vascular Nursing (see chapter 17, page 355) to get a decent description of the signs and symptoms. It's a long list, including chest pain, dyspnea, cough, sweats (diaphoresis), syncope, tachycardia, and cyanosis. —DR]

232. D. Rusty-brown color at ankles and calves.

▷Rumwell CB, McPharlin M: *Vascular Technology: An Illustrated Review*, 5th edition. Pasadena, CA, Davies Publishing, 2015, p 289.

233. C. Phlegmasia cerulea dolens.

▷Rumwell CB, McPharlin M: *Vascular Technology: An Illustrated Review*, 5th edition. Pasadena, CA, Davies Publishing, 2015, p 290.

234. D. Neither specific nor sensitive.

Deep venous thrombosis is famously difficult to call based on signs and symptoms, although again chronic unilateral edema is the single best predictor.

▷Dilley RB: The history and physical examination in vascular disease. In Bernstein EF (ed): *Vascular Diagnosis*, 4th edition. St. Louis, Mosby, 1993, p 12.

235. E. Thickening of toenails.

Thickening of the toenails is a sign of chronic arterial insufficiency.

▷Rumwell CB, McPharlin M: *Vascular Technology: An Illustrated Review*, 5th edition. Pasadena, CA, Davies Publishing, 2015, p 291.

236. C. Lesions are usually found on the lower third of the leg around the medial aspect of the ankle.

Venous ulcers are partially caused by the venous hypertension that exists during leg dependency. Venous ulceration typically occurs in the "gaiter area" around the medial aspect of the ankle, while arterial ulcers tend to show up on toes and feet. The pain associated with venous ulceration is usually mild. A venous ulcer, not due to arterial insufficiency, would be expected to ooze blood and to be able to exhibit granulation.

▷Rumwell CB, McPharlin M: *Vascular Technology: An Illustrated Review*, 5th edition. Pasadena, CA, Davies Publishing, 2015, pp 290–291.

237. D. Extensive left femoropopliteal deep venous thrombosis.

The massive edema suggests complete outflow obstruction and therefore a femoropopliteal thrombus. The obstruction must be proximal to the edema. The right knee pain is a bit of a red herring.

▷Pellerito JS, Polak JF: *Introduction to Vascular
Ultrasonography*, 6th edition. Philadelphia, Elsevier Saunders,
2012, p 346.

238. D. A hypoechoic mass in the shape of an egg at mid calf, thought to be a hematoma.

While a small number of patients will have the complication of thrombocytopenia (reduced platelets) with heparin treatment, a bleeding complication—hematoma—is the most likely answer here because of the pain closely associated with the administration of heparin.

▷Calaitges JG, Silver D: Antithrombotic therapy. In Rutherford
RB (ed): *Vascular Surgery*, 5th edition. Philadelphia, Saunders,
2000, p 437.

239. C. The popliteal vein is patent and the valves are incompetent.

This is the most likely finding, although chronic obstruction is a possibility. Congestive heart failure would cause bilateral—not unilateral—edema.

▷Moneta GL, Nehler MR, Porter JM: Pathophysiology of
chronic venous insufficiency. In Rutherford RB (ed): *Vascular
Surgery*, 5th edition. Philadelphia, Saunders, 2000, p 1985.

240. D. Ambulatory venous pressure.

Ambulatory venous pressure increases dramatically in chronic venous obstruction.

▷Criado E, Passman MA: Physiologic assessment of the
venous system. In Rutherford RB (ed): *Vascular Surgery*, 5th
edition. Philadelphia, Saunders, 2000, p 175.

241. C. Chronic venous insufficiency.

Brawny (toughened and swollen) changes almost always indicate venous insufficiency.

▷Rumwell CB, McPharlin M: *Vascular Technology: An
Illustrated Review*, 5th edition. Pasadena, CA, Davies
Publishing, 2015, pp 289–290.

242. B. Venous ulcers are usually not painful and are located cephalad to the foot.

Venous ulcers are usually not painful and located proximal to the medial malleolus cephalad to the foot. Venous ulcers are treated with Unna boots (compression system with medicated dressing); arterial ulcers are not.

▷Rumwell CB, McPharlin M: *Vascular Technology: An
Illustrated Review*, 5th edition. Pasadena, CA, Davies
Publishing, 2015, pp 290–291.

243. D. Tourniquet test.

The tourniquet test is primarily used to diagnose superficial venous incompetence. Note that Homans' sign is actually worse than useless as a diagnostic sign, since it gives the

illusion of doing something useful, when in fact it is neither sensitive nor specific for deep venous thrombosis. In fact, the edema is the only potentially useful physical finding here.

▷Rutherford RB: Initial patient evaluation: the vascular consultation. In Rutherford RB (ed): *Vascular Surgery*, 5th edition. Philadelphia, Saunders, 2000, p 9.

244. E. Tachypnea.

This is rapid respiration, frequently associated with pulmonary embolism.

▷Oliver MA: Clinical evaluation. In Talbot SR, Oliver MA: *Techniques of Venous Imaging.* Pasadena, CA, Davies Publishing, 1992, p 29.

245. D. Positive lower extremity venous ultrasound.

Ultrasonography is not a clinical sign but an exam. In any case, venous duplex is usually not a useful test for pulmonary embolism in the absence of lower extremity symptoms.

▷Oliver MA: Clinical evaluation. In Talbot SR, Oliver MA: *Techniques of Venous Imaging.* Pasadena, CA, Davies Publishing, 1992, p 29.

246. B. This statement—"It can best be diagnosed by photoplethysmography"—is NOT true of superficial thrombophlebitis in the leg.

Photoplethysmography is not a useful modality for this situation.

▷DePalma RG, Johnson Jr G: Superficial thrombophlebitis: diagnosis and management. In Rutherford RB (ed): *Vascular Surgery*, 5th edition. Philadelphia, Saunders, 2000, pp 1979–1981.

247. B. Pulmonary angiography.

This exam is not undertaken lightly, but it is the definitive test for pulmonary embolism.

▷Rumwell CB, McPharlin M: *Vascular Technology: An Illustrated Review*, 5th edition. Pasadena, CA, Davies Publishing, 2015, p 350.

248. C. A peroneal vein.

Since the calf veins are paired, continuous-wave (CW) flow signals may continue to sound normal in one branch even if the other branch is thrombosed. Additionally, peroneal veins are seldom assessed with handheld CW Doppler.

▷Rumwell CB, McPharlin M: *Vascular Technology: An Illustrated Review*, 5th edition. Pasadena, CA, Davies Publishing, 2015, pp 301–302.

249. D. Essentially normal venous refilling.

Venous incompetence is illustrated by refill times of less than 20 seconds. This well exceeds that refill time.

▷Rumwell CB, McPharlin M: *Vascular Technology: An Illustrated Review*, 5th edition. Pasadena, CA, Davies Publishing, 2015, pp 294–296.

250. D. Ultrasound imaging.

Ultrasound imaging may be useful because this patient has the classic symptoms of a Baker's cyst. The continuous CW Doppler signal would likely be the result of extrinsic compression of the vein.

▷Pellerito JS, Polak JF: *Introduction to Vascular Ultrasonography*, 6th edition. Philadelphia, Elsevier Saunders, 2012, pp 387, 392, 432–433.

251. A. Cessation of flow with proximal compression, resuming on release.

Augmentation with proximal compression or on release of distal compression indicates insufficiency.

▷Rumwell CB, McPharlin M: *Vascular Technology: An Illustrated Review*, 5th edition. Pasadena, CA, Davies Publishing, 2015, pp 303–306.

252. B. The Trendelenburg test.

This is a venerable test whose accuracy has been called into question.

▷Nicolaides AN: Basic aspects of peripheral venous testing. In Bernstein EF (ed): *Vascular Diagnosis*, 4th edition. St. Louis, Mosby, 1993, p 783.

253. D. Femoropopliteal and posterior tibial valvular insufficiency.

Proximal compression should not elicit flow signals if the valves are competent.

▷Rumwell CB, McPharlin M: *Vascular Technology: An Illustrated Review*, 5th edition. Pasadena, CA, Davies Publishing, 2015, p 305.

254. C. Superficial valvular insufficiency.

The tourniquet took the superficial system out of the picture, which returned the result to normal. Therefore, the superficial system caused the rapid refill.

▷Rumwell CB, McPharlin M: *Vascular Technology: An Illustrated Review*, 5th edition. Pasadena, CA, Davies Publishing, 2015, p 296.

255. E. This is a normal finding.

Femoral vein augmentation with gentle calf compression suggests probable patency between the two levels. This information can be helpful when the duplex scan is technically difficult.

▷Rumwell CB, McPharlin M: *Vascular Technology: An Illustrated Review*, 5th edition. Pasadena, CA, Davies Publishing, 2015, p 305.

256. D. Venous reflux.

Reflux may or may not be associated with deep venous thrombosis, but usually is a chronic condition found after the acute event.

257. A. Photoplethysmography.

PPG is not helpful in diagnosing acute thrombosis; it is used for diagnosing chronic venous insufficiency. IPG, SPG, and air plethysmography are all capacitance/outflow modalities, and their tracings look essentially the same.

▷Rumwell CB, McPharlin M: *Vascular Technology: An Illustrated Review*, 5th edition. Pasadena, CA, Davies Publishing, 2015, pp 293 ff.

[It is difficult to find all three modalities discussed in the same place. Pneumoplethysmography is often omitted, yet it may nowadays be the most common— among those still performing this exam—since it comes bundled with mini-lab types of instruments. These combine CW Doppler, arterial and venous plethysmography—both air type—and PPG.]

258. E. Are different from any of the above.

A low PRF (scale) setting is necessary for the slower flow in lower extremity veins.

259. E. All but C.

Inspiration diminishes venous flow from the lower extremities, because it increases pressure in the abdominal cavity (more pressure on the inferior vena cava). Proximal compression obviously diminishes venous outflow due to the pressure on the vein. The Valsalva maneuver should diminish venous flow everywhere in the body, as it increases both intraabdominal and intrathoracic pressure. Expiration decreases pressure in the abdomen, allowing venous outflow from the lower extremities to resume.

▷Rumwell CB, McPharlin M: *Vascular Technology: An Illustrated Review*, 5th edition. Pasadena, CA, Davies Publishing, 2015, pp 303–306.

260. C. Left-leg DVT.

The greatly increased flow in the left great saphenous vein suggests that it is acting as a major outflow collateral in the presence of deep vein thrombosis. The character of flow on

the right is within normal limits; it is common for flow in the great saphenous vein to be non-spontaneous. (This depends partly on whether the patient is warm or cool.) Sure, there could be less hemodynamically significant thrombosis on the right, but the saphenous flow does not suggest it.

261. C. Slows down or stops venous flow everywhere in the body.

Since the Valsalva maneuver increases pressure within both the thoracic and abdominal cavities, venous flow everywhere diminishes or ceases. This can help at times to distinguish pulsatile venous signals from arterial signals.

▷Rumwell CB, McPharlin M: *Vascular Technology: An Illustrated Review*, 5th edition. Pasadena, CA, Davies Publishing, 2015, pp 278–279.

262. B. Gaiety.

This would be a characteristic of a cheerful vascular technologist. The others are normal venous flow characteristics.

▷Rumwell CB, McPharlin M: *Vascular Technology: An Illustrated Review*, 5th edition. Pasadena, CA, Davies Publishing, 2015, pp 303–306.

263. B. Right iliac thrombosis.

If respiratory pressure changes are not transmitted to the lower extremity venous signals, the technologist should be suspicious of proximal obstruction.

▷Pellerito JS, Polak JF: *Introduction to Vascular Ultrasonography*, 6th edition. Philadelphia, Elsevier Saunders, 2012, p 346.

264. E. Answers A and C.

Semi–Fowler's position is raising the trunk and head, but not the knees (true Fowler's position includes raising the knees, which is what most hospital beds do when you raise the head). Reverse Trendelenburg's position is patient supine, head up, and feet down. A combination of these is usually used for venous duplex studies. Trendelenburg's position is patient supine, head down, and feet up—useful for pooling blood in the central circulation in hypotensive patients, but not for venous imaging or Doppler in the lower extremities. Supine, leg elevated is good for venous outflow plethysmography.

▷Rumwell CB, McPharlin M: *Vascular Technology: An Illustrated Review*, 5th edition. Pasadena, CA, Davies Publishing, 2015, p 303.

265. D. In a transverse plane without color flow.

The transverse plane allows careful visualization of the coapting walls as well as of multiple vessels. This part of the study is a gray-scale procedure; color flow should be left off to allow scrutiny of walls.

▷Talbot SR: Venous imaging technique. In Talbot SR, Oliver MA: *Techniques of Venous Imaging.* Pasadena, CA, Davies Publishing, 1992, p 66.

266. B. This finding is equivocal for significant valvular incompetence.

0.5 seconds of reflux is often cited as a threshold for calling incompetence, although some labs use a full second or longer.

▷Pellerito JS, Polak JF: *Introduction to Vascular Ultrasonography*, 6th edition. Philadelphia, Elsevier Saunders, 2012, pp 416–420.

267. A. Bright intraluminal echoes.

Bright intraluminal echoes are more compatible with organized, older thrombus.

▷Rumwell CB, McPharlin M: *Vascular Technology: An Illustrated Review*, 5th edition. Pasadena, CA, Davies Publishing, 2015, p 322.

268. E. Valvular incompetence cannot be assessed with CW Doppler.

You certainly can assess venous incompetence with hand-held CW. The other items do represent limitations.

▷Rumwell CB, McPharlin M: *Vascular Technology: An Illustrated Review*, 5th edition. Pasadena, CA, Davies Publishing, 2015, pp 301–302.

269. C. Chronic thrombosis.

The bright walls with a small recanalized lumen suggest an older episode.

▷Pellerito JS, Polak JF: *Introduction to Vascular Ultrasonography*, 6th edition. Philadelphia, Elsevier Saunders, 2012, pp 359–361.

270. B. Acute thrombosis.

These characteristics are consistent with (but do not guarantee) acute thrombus.

▷Pellerito JS, Polak JF: *Introduction to Vascular Ultrasonography*, 6th edition. Philadelphia, Elsevier Saunders, 2012, p 359.

271. E. Baker's cyst.

▷Pellerito JS, Polak JF: *Introduction to Vascular Ultrasonography*, 6th edition. Philadelphia, Elsevier Saunders, 2012, pp 432–433.

272. D. This suggests venous reflux.

This finding suggests significant venous valvular incompetence at this level.

▷Pellerito JS, Polak JF: *Introduction to Vascular Ultrasonography*, 6th edition. Philadelphia, Elsevier Saunders, 2012, pp 362–363.

273. C. The distal thigh.

This level, with its taut distal adductor muscles, is difficult to compress with the probe, but it need not be a problem. Some technologists scan more anteriorly, to use the quadriceps muscle as an acoustic window, and compress with the non–probe hand behind the thigh. Works well and doesn't hurt the patient.

▷Ridgway DA: *Introduction to Vascular Scanning*, 4th edition. Pasadena, CA, Davies Publishing, 2014, pp 199–200.

274. C. A remnant of recanalized old DVT.

This is a fairly common finding in patients with a history of deep venous thrombosis.

▷Pellerito JS, Polak JF: *Introduction to Vascular Ultrasonography*, 6th edition. Philadelphia, Elsevier Saunders, 2012, pp 359–361.

275. C. Congestive heart failure.

Anything that increases overall venous pressure, like congestive heart failure, can bring about pulsatility of the venous Doppler signals in the lower extremities.

▷Rumwell CB, McPharlin M: *Vascular Technology: An Illustrated Review*, 5th edition. Pasadena, CA, Davies Publishing, 2015, p 306.

276. B. Is within normal limits in a cold patient.

It is not uncommon to have nonspontaneous flow in either the posterior tibial or great saphenous veins, especially if the patient is nervous and/or cold and therefore vasoconstricted (i.e., less flow across to the venous side due to closed-down arterioles).

▷Talbot SR: Venous imaging technique. In Talbot SR, Oliver MA: *Techniques of Venous Imaging*. Pasadena, CA, Davies Publishing, 1992, p 60.

277. A. Suggests significant valvular incompetence.

The PPG tracing is a reflection of intravenous pressure. Following the dorsiflexions, which reduce intravenous pressure to a minimum, the return to original pressure should result

only from inflow from capillaries and therefore take at least 20 seconds. A rapid return like this one suggests that blood is refluxing because of valvular incompetence.

▷Rumwell CB, McPharlin M: *Vascular Technology: An Illustrated Review*, 5th edition. Pasadena, CA, Davies Publishing, 2015, p 296.

278. B. Suggests deep venous valvular incompetence.

The tourniquet eliminates the influence of the superficial system. Had the tracing reverted to normal with the tourniquet, the superficial system would then be implicated. In this case it is the deep veins— instead of or in addition to the superficial veins—that appear to be incompetent.

▷Rumwell CB, McPharlin M: *Vascular Technology: An Illustrated Review*, 5th edition. Pasadena, CA, Davies Publishing, 2015, p 296.

279. B. Valvular insufficiency.

Ascending venography defines the location and extent of venous obstruction. Descending venography identifies specific valvular incompetence. Answer choice E is a dirty trick: the IVC has no valves.

▷McKustch MA, Gloviczki P: Principles of venography. In Rutherford RB (ed): *Vascular Surgery*, 5th edition. Philadelphia, Saunders, 2000, p 305.

280. C. Invasive.

Contrast venography is a very sensitive and specific test, which has some hazard. It may be considered as a diagnostic tool in a patient with suspected deep venous thrombosis, especially in the event of equivocal noninvasive studies. Its major drawback is that it is invasive.

▷McKustch MA, Gloviczki P: Principles of venography. In Rutherford RB (ed): *Vascular Surgery*, 5th edition. Philadelphia, Saunders, 2000, p 303.

281. D. Dorsal vein on the foot.

▷McKustch MA, Gloviczki P: Principles of venography. In Rutherford RB (ed): *Vascular Surgery*, 5th edition. Philadelphia, Saunders, 2000, p 304.

282. A. Common femoral vein.

▷McKustch MA, Gloviczki P: Principles of venography. In Rutherford RB (ed): *Vascular Surgery*, 5th edition. Philadelphia, Saunders, 2000, p 306.

283. D. On an exam table tilted 60 degrees upright.

▷McKustch MA, Gloviczki P: Principles of venography. In
Rutherford RB (ed): *Vascular Surgery*, 5th edition.
Philadelphia, Saunders, 2000, p 304.

284. D. Iatrogenic CVA.

Actually, there is indeed a rare phenomenon called "paradoxical stroke," with DVT embolizing to the arterial side through a patent foramen ovale in the right atrial wall and thence to the brain. We often get a flurry of orders for venous exams on stroke patients from a resident who has just learned of this.

▷McKustch MA, Gloviczki P: Principles of venography. In
Rutherford RB (ed): *Vascular Surgery*, 5th edition.
Philadelphia, Saunders, 2000, p 309.

285. B. Area of no contrast, often with "railroad track" lines along walls.

This is a filling defect. The "string of pearls" sign is associated with fibromuscular hyperplasia. Well-developed collaterals would suggest a chronic rather than acute episode. Answer choice E does not address the deep system.

▷Hull RD, Raskob GE, Hirsh J: Comparative value of tests for
the diagnosis of venous thrombosis. In Bernstein EF (ed):
Vascular Diagnosis, 4th edition. St. Louis, Mosby, 1993, p 849.

286. D. Pulmonary angiography.

(Astoundingly, I can find no discussion of pulmonary angiography in any of our core references. Diagnosis of pulmonary embolism is still frequently fuzzy: V/Q scans are often equivocal, and there is confusion as to whether it is useful to order a DVT study as an adjunctive test. So I'm surprised to see so little on the subject in the big vascular diagnostic texts. You'll have to trust me. —DR)

287. B. V/Q scan.

▷Rumwell CB, McPharlin M: *Vascular Technology: An
Illustrated Review*, 5th edition. Pasadena, CA, Davies
Publishing, 2015, p 334.

288. E. Can cause thrombocytopenia.

Heparin is a protein. As such, it can activate antibodies in a sensitized individual. It affects the partial thromboplastin time, but not the prothrombin time. It has no direct actions on clots once they are formed. Protamine is used to reverse the effects of heparin. The drug has a significant complication rate and can produce thrombocytopenia (diminished blood platelet count).

▷Calaitges JG, Silver D: Antithrombotic therapy. In Rutherford
RB (ed): *Vascular Surgery*, 5th edition. Philadelphia, Saunders,
2000, p 437.

289. C. A and B above.

Elevation and surgical support hose both tend to decrease venous hypertension and therefore increase the chances for ulcer healing and decrease pain and other problems of chronic venous insufficiency.

▷Moneta GL, Porter JM: Nonoperative treatment of chronic venous insufficiency. In Rutherford RB (ed): *Vascular Surgery*, 5th edition. Philadelphia, Saunders, 2000, p 1999.

290. C. Decreased activated partial thromboplastin time.

This would be expected to increase, and in any case the increase isn't a complication but a desired result for therapy.

▷Calaitges JG, Silver D: Antithrombotic therapy. In Rutherford RB (ed): *Vascular Surgery*, 5th edition. Philadelphia, Saunders, 2000, p 442.

291. E. Sodium warfarin.

Sodium warfarin or coumadin is the drug of choice for long-term anticoagulation.

▷Calaitges JG, Silver D: Antithrombotic therapy. In Rutherford RB (ed): *Vascular Surgery*, 5th edition. Philadelphia, Saunders, 2000, p 438.

292. E. The Jones wire arch.

The Jones wire arch is not a method of interrupting the vena cava. The Greenfield is the oldest and most widely used design. Nitinol is a nickel-titanium alloy that can be straightened for insertion, then resumes its shape on contact with the warmth of blood flow.

▷Greenfield LJ: Caval interruption procedures. In Rutherford RB (ed): *Vascular Surgery*, 5th edition. Philadelphia, Saunders, 2000, p 1969 ff.

293. E. Night cramps.

Night cramps usually are not a symptom of venous disease (or arterial, for that matter). Diminished cardiac output is a possible complication to ligation of the vena cava. The other symptoms would be secondary to significant caval obstruction (either ligation or a full filter) and consequently elevated venous pressures.

▷Greenfield LJ: Caval interruption procedures. In Rutherford RB (ed): *Vascular Surgery*, 5th edition. Philadelphia, Saunders, 2000, p 1968.

294. A. Heparin.

Since the age of deep vein thrombosis is unknown, heparin remains the drug of choice to initiate treatment.

▷Calaitges JG, Silver D: Antithrombotic therapy. In Rutherford RB (ed): *Vascular Surgery*, 5th edition. Philadelphia, Saunders, 2000, p 443.

PERIPHERAL ARTERIAL DISEASE

295. E. Saccular.

"Saccular" describes a shape of aneurysm, not the etiology.

▷Glickman BS, Rehm JP, Baxter BT: Arterial aneurysms: etiologic considerations. In Rutherford RB (ed): *Vascular Surgery*, 5th edition. Philadelphia, Saunders, 2000, p 374.

296. B. Degenerative origin.

Most aneurysms, especially in the abdominal aorta, are degenerative because of atherosclerosis.

▷Glickman BS, Rehm JP, Baxter BT: Arterial aneurysms: etiologic considerations. In Rutherford RB (ed): *Vascular Surgery*, 5th edition. Philadelphia, Saunders, 2000, p 377.

297. C. Takayasu's arteritis.

▷Giordano JM, Hoffman GS: Takayasu's disease: nonspecific aortoarteritis. In Rutherford RB (ed): *Vascular Surgery*, 5th edition. Philadelphia, Saunders, 2000, p 364 ff.

298. B. The heart.

The heart is the source of 80–90% of peripheral arterial embolic activity in the extremities. The other common source of peripheral arterial emboli is aneurysmal mural thrombus, especially in the aorta, iliac, femoral, and popliteal arteries. On the other hand, the most common source of <u>cerebrovascular</u> embolic activity is atherosclerotic carotid disease.

▷Greenberg RK, Ouriel K: Arterial thromboembolism. In Rutherford RB (ed): *Vascular Surgery*, 5th edition. Philadelphia, Saunders, 2000, p 822.

299. D. Congenital arterial wall weakness.

Although aneurysmal disorders may be related to trauma, congenital weakness and atherosclerosis are the most common causes of aneurysmal disease.

▷Zarins CK, Glagov S: Artery wall pathology in atherosclerosis. In Rutherford RB (ed): *Vascular Surgery*, 5th edition. Philadelphia, Saunders, 2000, p 328.

300. B. Thromboangiitis obliterans.

Thromboangiitis obliterans, also known as Buerger's disease, is usually seen in young males with a pronounced addiction to cigarette smoking. As legend has it, this addiction is so severe that patients with stumps for hands may continue to smoke.

▷Olin JW: Thromboangiitis obliterans (Buerger's disease). In Rutherford RB (ed): *Vascular Surgery*, 5th edition. Philadelphia, Saunders, 2000, p 350 ff.

301. B. Compartment syndrome.

▷Johansen KH, Watson JC: Compartment syndrome: pathophysiology, recognition, and management. In Rutherford RB (ed): *Vascular Surgery*, 5th edition. Philadelphia, Saunders, 2000, p 902.

302. C. Foot lesions.

Foot lesions are often found in diabetic patients with peripheral neuropathy (with or without peripheral atherosclerosis).

▷Seabrook GR, Towne JB: Management of foot lesions in the diabetic patient. In Rutherford RB (ed): *Vascular Surgery*, 5th edition. Philadelphia, Saunders, 2000, p 1093.

303. E. 80%.

30–50% of patients with AAA rupture die before reaching a hospital, and operative mortality is 40–50%. These facts highlight the desirability of catching abdominal aortic aneurysms before they rupture.

▷Cronenwett JL, Krupski WC, Rutherford RB: Abdominal aortic and iliac aneurysms. In Rutherford RB (ed): *Vascular Surgery*, 5th edition. Philadelphia, Saunders, 2000, p 1246.

304. B. This statement about smoking—"It increases the oxygen-carrying capacity of blood"—is false.

Carbon monoxide is one of many byproducts of smoking. Carbon monoxide decreases the oxygen-carrying ability of red blood cells. Smoking is really, really bad for you.

▷Sidawy AN, Mitchell ME: Basic considerations of the arterial wall. In Rutherford RB (ed): *Vascular Surgery*, 5th edition. Philadelphia, Saunders, 2000, p 69.

305. B. The arterial segment beginning in Hunter's canal.

Another name for Hunter's canal is the adductor canal, located in the mid-to-lower thigh. This is the most common site of atherosclerotic involvement in the lower extremities.

▷Zwiebel WJ: *Introduction to Vascular Ultrasonography*, 5th edition. Philadelphia, Elsevier Saunders, 2005, p 253.

▷Rumwell CB, McPharlin M: *Vascular Technology: An Illustrated Review*, 5th edition. Pasadena, CA, Davies Publishing, 2015, p 47.

306. G. B, C, and D.

Popliteal aneurysms have a very low risk of rupture but a high risk of embolization or thrombosis leading to loss of limb. There are occasional venous or neurologic symptoms due to size. About 50–70% of patients with a popliteal aneurysm have them bilaterally. Additionally, there is a high rate (about 40–50%) of coexisting abdominal aortic aneurysm in these patients. Claudication is a rare symptom and when present is the result of coexistent stenosis, not the aneurysmal process.

▷Graham LM: Femoral and popliteal aneurysms. In Rutherford RB (ed): *Vascular Surgery*, 5th edition. Philadelphia, Saunders, 2000, p 1351.

307. E. Most prerupture AAAs are discovered because of abdominal symptoms or distal emboli.

AAAs rarely extend above the renal arteries. The "gold standard" test has been B-mode ultrasound, although CT scanning is gaining popularity. Arteriograms are obtained prior to operation by some surgeons but may be falsely negative for diagnosing the aneurysm because of laminated clot within the lumen. Most aneurysms are discovered on routine physical examination while the patient is asymptomatic.

▷Cronenwett JL, Krupski WC, Rutherford RB: Abdominal aortic and iliac aneurysms. In Rutherford RB (ed): *Vascular Surgery*, 5th edition. Philadelphia, Saunders, 2000, p 1251.

308. B. Greater than 4 times the risk in the general population.

Diabetes is a significant risk factor in lower extremity arterial disease.

▷Hiatt WR, Cooke JP: Atherogenesis and the medical management of atherosclerosis. In Rutherford RB (ed): *Vascular Surgery*, 5th edition. Philadelphia, Saunders, 2000, p 335.

309. A. Hypolipidemia.

Hypolipidemia is not a risk factor for any vascular occlusive disease.

▷Rumwell CB, McPharlin M: *Vascular Technology: An Illustrated Review*, 5th edition. Pasadena, CA, Davies Publishing, 2015, pp 46–47.

310. B. Abdominal aortic aneurysm.

Abdominal aortic aneurysm (particularly if rupturing) often present with back, abdominal, or flank pain.

▷Cronenwett JL, Krupski WC, Rutherford RB: Abdominal aortic and iliac aneurysms. In Rutherford RB (ed): *Vascular Surgery*, 5th edition. Philadelphia, Saunders, 2000, p 1251.

311. D. Young women.

Takayasu's arteritis is usually found in young women in the second or third decade of life. It occurs most frequently in Asian women.

▷Giordano JM, Hoffman GS: Takayasu's disease: nonspecific aortoarteritis. In Rutherford RB (ed): *Vascular Surgery*, 5th edition. Philadelphia, Saunders, 2000, p 364.

312. E. A, B, and D.

Skin pigmentation changes are usually found in patients with chronic venous disease. Dependent rubor as well as thickening of the toenails and hair loss is indicative of chronic arterial insufficiency.

▷Rumwell CB, McPharlin M: *Vascular Technology: An Illustrated Review*, 5th edition. Pasadena, CA, Davies Publishing, 2015, p 54.

313. A. Blue color of tissue due to ischemia.

▷Rumwell CB, McPharlin M: *Vascular Technology: An Illustrated Review*, 5th edition. Pasadena, CA, Davies Publishing, 2015, p 290.

314. A.-5.   B.-3.   C.-1.   D.-4.   E.-2.

Some of this is sorted out by elimination. DVT (2) is the obvious choice for edema. A bruit cannot result from total occlusion, which eliminates 1, 3, and 4, leaving iliac artery stenosis (5). There is only aortoiliac/SFA occlusion (1) left to account for the foot rubor; the iliac artery stenosis is unlikely to produce such an advanced symptom anyway. Weakness of the right side most likely results from the left carotid occlusion (4), leaving the subclavian artery occlusion (3) to account for the absent pulse. Didn't like this question? Don't worry, the registry exam doesn't use this format.

315. A. Elevation pallor, dependent rubor.

Elevation creates negative hydrostatic pressure, decreasing lower extremity perfusion, so the foot turns cadaverously pale. Having the patient then dangle the leg restores perfusion, and the foot turns very red.

▷Rumwell CB, McPharlin M: *Vascular Technology: An Illustrated Review*, 5th edition. Pasadena, CA, Davies Publishing, 2015, p 55.

316. B. Cramping pain in the calf, thigh, or buttocks with exercise and relieved by rest.

▷Rumwell CB, McPharlin M: *Vascular Technology: An Illustrated Review*, 5th edition. Pasadena, CA, Davies Publishing, 2015, pp 45–46.

317. C. Foot pain while in a horizontal position relieved by standing or dangling the foot in a dependent position.

   Rest pain almost always occurs at night and is relieved by placing the leg in a dependent position or by exercise, which increases cardiac output and thereby blood flow to the periphery.

▷Rumwell CB, McPharlin M: *Vascular Technology: An Illustrated Review*, 5th edition. Pasadena, CA, Davies Publishing, 2015, p 46.

318. E. All of the above.

   Since the location of the ulcers and gangrene is not specified, any of the causes may be implicated.

319. E. Pedal ulcer.

   A pedal ulcer would take a bit more time to develop and is more characteristic of chronic rather than acute occlusion. The other of those "five Ps" of acute occlusion is pain. "Polar" (cold extremity—a strenuous effort to use the letter P for all of the symptoms) is sometimes added.

▷Rumwell CB, McPharlin M: *Vascular Technology: An Illustrated Review*, 5th edition. Pasadena, CA, Davies Publishing, 2015, p 46.

320. E. All except D.

   Pigmentation is a characteristic symptom of venous rather than arterial insufficiency.

▷Rumwell CB, McPharlin M: *Vascular Technology: An Illustrated Review*, 5th edition. Pasadena, CA, Davies Publishing, 2015, pp 54–55.

321. E. These symptoms are not typical of vascular disease.

   These symptoms do not suggest claudication, symptoms of which are quite consistent. The pain associated with claudication is a muscle fatigue due to anoxia brought on by exercise. Claudication usually does not occur within moments of starting to walk, and, if it does, the distance one can walk is extremely limited.

▷Rutherford RB: Initial patient evaluation: the vascular consultation. In Rutherford RB (ed): *Vascular Surgery*, 5th edition. Philadelphia, Saunders, 2000, p 3.

322. A. An infection.

Diabetic foot infections can happen with or without peripheral vascular disease.

▷Seabrook GR, Towne JB: Management of foot lesions in the
diabetic patient. In Rutherford RB (ed): *Vascular Surgery*, 5th
edition. Philadelphia, Saunders, 2000, p 1094.

323. C. A pseudoaneurysm of the femoral artery.

*Femoral artery pseudoaneurysms are often found after catheterization. Hematomas after
cardiac catheterization are also frequent but usually do not pulsate.*

▷Rumwell CB, McPharlin M: *Vascular Technology: An
Illustrated Review*, 5th edition. Pasadena, CA, Davies
Publishing, 2015, pp 48–50.

324. C. Claudication.

*All of the rest of the symptoms generally come with acute or late chronic occlusive changes
(except for swelling, which often accompanies venous thrombosis).*

▷Rumwell CB, McPharlin M: *Vascular Technology: An
Illustrated Review*, 5th edition. Pasadena, CA, Davies
Publishing, 2015, p 45.

325. E. Progressive claudication.

*Progressive claudication is usually associated with slow progression of atherosclerosis,
not with embolization.*

▷Rumwell CB, McPharlin M: *Vascular Technology: An
Illustrated Review*, 5th edition. Pasadena, CA, Davies
Publishing, 2015, pp 45–46.

326. B. Pain at night in the forefoot or foot that may go away with leg dependency.

*Nocturnal forefoot pain relieved by dependency or exercise is the most common complaint
of patients with rest pain.*

▷Rumwell CB, McPharlin M: *Vascular Technology: An
Illustrated Review*, 5th edition. Pasadena, CA, Davies
Publishing, 2015, p 46.

327. D. Claudication.

*Claudication may be experienced months or years prior to an acute arterial occlusion, or it
may not be felt at all prior to the episode. The other symptoms are consistent with an acute
event.*

▷Rumwell CB, McPharlin M: *Vascular Technology: An
Illustrated Review*, 5th edition. Pasadena, CA, Davies
Publishing, 2015, p 46.

328. B. Very painful and commonly located distally over the dorsum of the foot.

An ulcer found above the medial malleolus is most likely venous in origin.

▷Rumwell CB, McPharlin M: *Vascular Technology: An
Illustrated Review*, 5th edition. Pasadena, CA, Davies
Publishing, 2015, p 54.

329. D. Dorsum of foot.

▷Carter SA: Clinical problems in peripheral arterial disease: is
the clinical diagnosis adequate. In Bernstein EF (ed): Vascular
Diagnosis, 4th edition. St. Louis, Mosby, 1993, p 475.

330. E. A thrill.

A thrill is the palpable manifestation of a bruit. Both are caused by wall vibration.

▷Rumwell CB, McPharlin M: *Vascular Technology: An
Illustrated Review*, 5th edition. Pasadena, CA, Davies
Publishing, 2015, p 56.

331. D. Red skin color.

*Examples are the cherry-red color of digits in a Raynaud's patient when the digital arteries
reopen after prolonged spasm, or the bright red foot on dependency after elevation in a
patient with advanced arterial occlusive disease.*

▷Rumwell CB, McPharlin M: *Vascular Technology: An
Illustrated Review*, 5th edition. Pasadena, CA, Davies
Publishing, 2015, p 54.

332. C. On toes and distal foot.

▷Rutherford RB: Initial patient evaluation: the vascular
consultation. In Rutherford RB (ed): *Vascular Surgery*, 5th
edition. Philadelphia, Saunders, 2000, p 10.

333. C. Advanced ischemia.

*Capillary blush usually is seen after 1–2 seconds. In patients with significant ischemia, it
may be delayed for many seconds.*

▷Rumwell CB, McPharlin M: *Vascular Technology: An
Illustrated Review*, 5th edition. Pasadena, CA, Davies
Publishing, 2015, p 54.

▷Rutherford RB: Initial patient evaluation: the vascular
consultation. In Rutherford RB (ed): *Vascular Surgery*, 5th
edition. Philadelphia, Saunders, 2000, p 9.

334. D. Pitting edema.

*True pitting edema is usually a symptom of systemic disease (such as CHF), chronic
venous disease, or lymphedema.*

▷Rutherford RB: Initial patient evaluation: the vascular consultation. In Rutherford RB (ed): *Vascular Surgery*, 5th edition. Philadelphia, Saunders, 2000, p 10.

335. E. Peroneal.

▷Rumwell CB, McPharlin M: *Vascular Technology: An Illustrated Review*, 5th edition. Pasadena, CA, Davies Publishing, 2015, p 56.

336. B. Cannot rule out significant stenosis at that level.

Bruits heard on physical examination are useful: Although the absence of a bruit does not rule out significant arterial obstruction, the presence of a bruit does suggest stenosis.

▷Rumwell CB, McPharlin M: *Vascular Technology: An Illustrated Review*, 5th edition. Pasadena, CA, Davies Publishing, 2015, p 56.

337. B. Presence of a bruit may be the first indication of arterial disease.

Again, hearing a bruit is more significant than not hearing one.

338. E. All of the above.

▷Johansen KH, Watson JC: Compartment syndrome: pathophysiology, recognition, and management. In Rutherford RB (ed): *Vascular Surgery*, 5th edition. Philadelphia, Saunders, 2000, p 903.

339. A. Popliteal artery entrapment.

Popliteal artery entrapment is the most common cause of unilateral claudication in a young person.

▷Rumwell CB, McPharlin M: *Vascular Technology: An Illustrated Review*, 5th edition. Pasadena, CA, Davies Publishing, 2015, pp 169–170.

340. B. Raynaud's phenomenon.

Raynaud's phenomenon causes prolonged digital pallor or cyanosis, followed by rubor on reperfusion.

▷Rumwell CB, McPharlin M: *Vascular Technology: An Illustrated Review*, 5th edition. Pasadena, CA, Davies Publishing, 2015, p 52.

341. D. Peak systolic to peak end diastolic velocity divided by mean velocity.

This is also known as Gosling's pulsatility index. This index is used mostly with continuous-wave Doppler or transcranial Doppler and increases with increased distal resistance. It is independent of the Doppler angle.

▷Rumwell CB, McPharlin M: *Vascular Technology: An Illustrated Review*, 5th edition. Pasadena, CA, Davies Publishing, 2015, p 67.

▷Johnston KW: Processing continuous wave Doppler signals and analysis of peripheral arterial waveforms: problems and solutions. In Bernstein EF (ed): *Vascular Diagnosis*, 4th edition. St. Louis, Mosby, 1993, p 152.

342. B. There is pressure drop distal to the obstructed segment after exercise.

Peripheral flow is generally maintained at rest by compensatory vasodilatation distally. Exercise causes pronounced vasodilatation, greatly increasing flow. Although claudicators usually have a reduced resting pressure, they can sometimes have equivocal or even essentially normal ABIs at rest. Thus some form of challenge (exercise or postocclusive reactive hyperemia) might be required to provoke a pressure drop.

▷Sumner DS: Essential hemodynamic principles. In Rutherford RB (ed): *Vascular Surgery*, 5th edition. Philadelphia, Saunders, 2000, p 84.

343. A. An increase in peripheral resistance.

This question refers to the effects of the arterial pressure wave, an energy wave that travels throughout the arterial tree with each systolic ejection from the heart. This energy is reflected primarily from the arterioles, and the amount of reflection obviously depends on the vasomotor state. A decrease in peripheral resistance and/or vasodilation will cause a decrease in pulse amplitude, since less of the pressure-wave energy is reflected proximally. An increase of distal resistance (vasoconstriction) reflects more of the pressure-wave energy proximally. This reflected energy sums with existing energy in the proximal arteries to increase pulsatility and pressure.

▷Sumner DS: Essential hemodynamic principles. In Rutherford RB (ed): *Vascular Surgery*, 5th edition. Philadelphia, Saunders, 2000, p 85 ff.

344. B. Hyperemia is prolonged in obstructed limbs in comparison to limbs with no obstruction.

Hyperemia is prolonged in patients with significant obstruction. Cardiac output is partly a function of how much blood the peripheral circulation is willing to accept. Decreased peripheral resistance, such as after reactive hyperemia or exercise, would tend to increase cardiac output.

▷Pellerito JS, Polak JF:: *Introduction to Vascular Ultrasonography*, 6th edition. Philadelphia, Elsevier Saunders, 2012, pp 256–257.

345. C. In the range of 0.5–0.9.

This is the traditional answer, but lots of patients with ABIs as low as 0.3 are still claudicators—that is, they have not reached the rest-pain stage.

▷Rumwell CB, McPharlin M: *Vascular Technology: An Illustrated Review*, 5th edition. Pasadena, CA, Davies Publishing, 2015, p 75.

346. D. Ankle pressure by the higher brachial pressure.

▷Rumwell CB, McPharlin M: *Vascular Technology: An Illustrated Review*, 5th edition. Pasadena, CA, Davies Publishing, 2015, p 74.

347. D. >50% SFA stenosis.

A common criterion for lower extremity arteries (and a good rule of thumb in any arteries): A stenotic velocity that accelerates to double that of the prestenotic velocity suggests >50% stenosis.

▷Rumwell CB, McPharlin M: *Vascular Technology: An Illustrated Review*, 5th edition. Pasadena, CA, Davies Publishing, 2015, pp 233–236.

348. A. Right femoral artery obstruction.

The obstruction must be proximal to the high-thigh cuff, but not as far proximal as the aortic segment, since the left side is within normal limits. (Right iliac artery obstruction is a possibility, of course, but is not one of the choices here.)

▷Zwiebel WJ: *Introduction to Vascular Ultrasonography*, 5th edition. Philadelphia, Elsevier Saunders, 2005, p 271.

349. C. A pressure transducer monitoring cuff pressure over a limb.

The electrode bands are used in impedance plethysmography, the photocells are used in photoplethysmography, the mercury-filled silastic tube is used in strain-gauge plethysmography, and the big air cuff is used in APG (air plethysmography, the modality designed specifically for testing of chronic venous insufficiency).

▷Rumwell CB, McPharlin M: *Vascular Technology: An Illustrated Review*, 5th edition. Pasadena, CA, Davies Publishing, 2015, pp 99–103.

350. D. Alternately compressing the radial and ulnar arteries while listening for changes in the digital artery signal.

While B and C are partly true, you must compress both arteries (alternately) to see whether flow persists to the hand.

▷Rumwell CB, McPharlin M: *Vascular Technology: An Illustrated Review*, 5th edition. Pasadena, CA, Davies Publishing, 2015, pp 84–87.

351. E. A and C.

Subclavian steal is a more proximal problem. Evaluation of the palmar arch is useful both before and after the placement of an arteriovenous arm shunt or for digital disease. (A careful Allen test is now being used as well before harvest of the radial artery for coronary artery bypass.)

▷Rumwell CB, McPharlin M: *Vascular Technology: An Illustrated Review*, 5th edition. Pasadena, CA, Davies Publishing, 2015, pp 84–85.

352. C. A common femoral or superficial femoral artery waveform.

The upper extremity is a high-resistance system similar to the legs. Although flow reversal is usually not as dramatic as in the lower extremities, there will be the same type of Doppler waveform as in other high-resistance beds.

▷Rumwell CB, McPharlin M: *Vascular Technology: An Illustrated Review*, 5th edition. Pasadena, CA, Davies Publishing, 2015, p 66.

353. A. This velocity may be normal for this graft.

The 45 cm/sec threshold for graft failure has had wide circulation, but other factors may make it invalid. For example, the distal end of the reversed vein graft, being larger in diameter, might be expected to have velocities that are lower than those at the proximal end. The important finding would be significant changes from the baseline exam. Gibson et al. (Journal of Vascular Surgery 33:24–31, 2001) suggest criteria for diagnosing impending graft failure that include mean graft velocity.

▷Rumwell CB, McPharlin M: *Vascular Technology: An Illustrated Review*, 5th edition. Pasadena, CA, Davies Publishing, 2015, p 41.

354. E. Distal turbulence.

▷Rumwell CB, McPharlin M: *Vascular Technology: An Illustrated Review*, 5th edition. Pasadena, CA, Davies Publishing, 2015, pp 39–41.

355. C. Extremity arteries at rest.

The renal and internal carotid arteries supply low-resistance vascular beds, which bring about increased forward flow during diastole. During exercise, peripheral resistance decreases, diminishing or eliminating diastolic reversal. Diastolic flow reversal is not a characteristic of venous flow.

▷Pellerito JS, Polak JF: *Introduction to Vascular Ultrasonography*, 6th edition. Philadelphia, Elsevier Saunders, 2012, pp 10–11.

356. B. The peripheral resistance is usually lower in the upper extremity.

A brachial artery waveform without flow reversal is a common finding.

▷Rumwell CB, McPharlin M: *Vascular Technology: An Illustrated Review*, 5th edition. Pasadena, CA, Davies Publishing, 2015, p 66.

357. C. Popliteal entrapment.

Claudication-like symptoms in a young person, especially a muscular male, are likely due to popliteal entrapment. Atherosclerotic obstruction is very unlikely; Compartment syndrome generally follows injury and/or reperfusion. Coarctation would cause symptoms in both lower extremities. The symptoms of deep venous thrombosis are very different and would not cause a decrease in arterial pressure.

▷Rumwell CB, McPharlin M: *Vascular Technology: An Illustrated Review*, 5th edition. Pasadena, CA, Davies Publishing, 2015, pp 169–170.

358. D. Anterior tibial artery.

The significant drop is from low thigh to anterior tibial; the drop from low thigh to posterior tibial is within normal limits. This information localizes the obstruction to the proximal anterior tibial segment (i.e., proximal to the below-knee cuff).

▷Rumwell CB, McPharlin M: *Vascular Technology: An Illustrated Review*, 5th edition. Pasadena, CA, Davies Publishing, 2015, pp 75–76.

359. A. SFA obstruction.

The low-thigh reading of 144 mmHg is a "reverse gradient," usually an artifactual problem: poor cuff application, cuff too narrow, even a partially incompressible artery due to medial calcification. SFA obstruction would be expected to decrease the low-thigh pressure.

▷Rumwell CB, McPharlin M: *Vascular Technology: An Illustrated Review*, 5th edition. Pasadena, CA, Davies Publishing, 2015, pp 70–72.

360. B. B-mode ultrasound.

B-mode ultrasound does not provide hemodynamic information about the arteries, only images. (No, you can't try to watch the wall pulsation. Just forget it.) All other cited methods can be and have been used to monitor pulses for pressure measurement.

▷Carter SA: Role of pressure measurements. In Bernstein EF (ed): *Vascular Diagnosis*, 4th edition. St. Louis, Mosby, 1993, p 486.

361. C. Suggests interference from venous flow.

Since continuous-wave analog Doppler displays net or average frequency shifts (i.e., velocities) of all flow intersecting the beam, venous flow can interfere with your efforts to get a clear arterial tracing on paper.

▷Strandness Jr DE: Doppler ultrasonic techniques in vascular disease. In Bernstein EF (ed): *Vascular Diagnosis*, 4th edition. St. Louis, Mosby, 1993, p 69.

362. C. Speed is varied during cardiac testing.

The standard cardiac treadmill protocol aims to increase the heart rate to a specific target level. This is accomplished by increasing the speed and elevation of the treadmill at specific time intervals during the examination. Treadmill testing for claudication generally uses one unvarying speed and elevation. Both types of exam include blood pressure monitoring, as well as observation by technologists. There is some cardiac risk associated with claudication testing.

▷Rumwell CB, McPharlin M: *Vascular Technology: An Illustrated Review*, 5th edition. Pasadena, CA, Davies Publishing, 2015, pp 77–78.

363. E. Isolated profunda femoral artery disease.

Any lesion proximal to the cuff can cause an abnormally low high-thigh pressure. In addition, the equivalent of a common femoral artery lesion, by the presence of disease in both the superficial femoral and profunda arteries, can likewise lower the high-thigh pressure. However, isolated profunda lesions are usually not detectable by pressure changes.

▷Pellerito JS, Polak JF: *Introduction to Vascular Ultrasonography*, 6th edition. Philadelphia, Elsevier Saunders, 2012, p 254.

364. B. Angina.

The classic description of angina is chest pain, sometimes with radiation to the jaw and/or arm. However, some patients do not have the chest pain component, but do have the other symptoms. This patient must be assumed to have angina until proven otherwise.

365. B. The dorsalis pedis artery pressure should be used to calculate the ankle/brachial index.

The higher ankle pressure is used to calculate the index. There may be disease limited to the calf arteries, but there may also be disease above the knee; this information alone does not allow us to say which is the case. Whereas the two branches of the tibioperoneal trunk have equal pressures, each vessel may independently be diseased, and disease in the trunk cannot be diagnosed with this information.

▷Baker JD: The vascular laboratory. In Rutherford RB (ed): *Vascular Surgery*, 5th edition. Philadelphia, Saunders, 2000, p 136.

366. A. Aortoiliac obstruction.

Since the left high-thigh pressure is within normal limits, the aortic segment cannot be included in the diagnosis of obstruction.

367. B. 2–3 cm.

▷Rumwell CB, McPharlin M: *Vascular Technology: An Illustrated Review*, 5th edition. Pasadena, CA, Davies Publishing, 2015, p 141.

368. C. Is higher than expected.

Due to the physical examination this pressure is much higher than suggested and would lead one to think that the pressures might be artificially higher than normal, perhaps due to calcification. Patients with rest pain usually have pressures less than 60 mmHg and ABI < 0.30.

▷Pellerito JS, Polak JF: *Introduction to Vascular Ultrasonography*, 6th edition. Philadelphia, Elsevier Saunders, 2012, p 252.

369. B. Erroneous due to probable arterial calcification.

The result is likely due to calcified and incompressible arteries. This is very common in diabetic patients, so answer choice A is quite possible but not proven.

▷Rumwell CB, McPharlin M: *Vascular Technology: An Illustrated Review*, 5th edition. Pasadena, CA, Davies Publishing, 2015, p 75.

370. C. Is an incomplete evaluation of this patient.

Arterial pressures at rest may be in the normal range, with only stress bringing out the abnormalities. To completely evaluate this patient, the circulation must be challenged by exercise or reactive hyperemia. Until that test is performed, significant vascular disease cannot be ruled out.

▷Zierler RE, Sumner DS: Physiologic assessment of peripheral arterial occlusive disease. In Rutherford RB (ed): *Vascular Surgery*, 5th edition. Philadelphia, Saunders, 2000, p 148.

▷Carter SA: Role of pressure measurements. In Bernstein EF (ed): *Vascular Diagnosis*, 4th edition. St. Louis, Mosby, 1993, p 491.

371. D. Are typical for patients with claudication.

One cannot call occlusion vs. stenosis based on this information. These decreases suggest mild disease on the left and more pronounced disease on the right, typical findings in a claudicating patient.

▷Strandness Jr DE, Zierler RE: Exercise ankle pressure measurements in arterial disease. In Bernstein EF (ed): *Vascular Diagnosis*, 4th edition. St. Louis, Mosby, 1993, p 552.

372. A. 0.50 (90/180).

You use the higher brachial pressure to calculate the index.

▷Rumwell CB, McPharlin M: *Vascular Technology: An Illustrated Review*, 5th edition. Pasadena, CA, Davies Publishing, 2015, p 74.

373. D. This statement—"The patient has renovascular hypertension"—is NOT true.

This patient has bilateral lower extremity obstructive disease based on these pressures and indices. There appears also to be obstruction proximal to the left brachial cuff (60 mmHg gradient compared to right arm); this is usually caused by subclavian disease. The patient has hypertension (systemic pressure of 180 mmHg), but the reason for this finding cannot be ascertained from this exam. Renovascular hypertension is only one cause of this problem, and is responsible for 3–5% of hypertension cases.

▷Rumwell CB, McPharlin M: *Vascular Technology: An Illustrated Review*, 5th edition. Pasadena, CA, Davies Publishing, 2015, p 74.

▷Zwiebel WJ: *Introduction to Vascular Ultrasonography*, 5th edition. Philadelphia, Elsevier Saunders, 2005, pp 616–621.

374. G. A, B, and C.

Since the patient complains of pain in the right leg that is worse than the left, he is ipso facto symptomatically worse in the right leg. There is a drop in pressure in both legs; therefore, there is vascular disease in both legs. As to the symptoms, they do not follow the usual pattern of claudication; they do not progress with the exercise. Therefore, it is likely that at least most of the pain is not vascular in origin.

▷Rutherford RB: Initial patient evaluation: the vascular consultation. In Rutherford RB (ed): *Vascular Surgery*, 5th edition. Philadelphia, Saunders, 2000, p 3.

375. F. A and B.

Pressure in both legs is reduced, both at rest and after exercise, and the magnitude of the pressure decrease is greater on the left than on the right, suggesting more severe disease on that side. The level of disease cannot be ascertained from these data. The patient should give essentially the same results after recovery. The lack of blood pressure increase in the arm may mean only a relatively healthy systemic-pressure response to exercise. (Answer

choice I is possible, but it is not the <u>best</u> answer. The registry exam will not offer this many choices.)

▷Zierler RE, Sumner DS: Physiologic assessment of peripheral arterial occlusive disease. In Rutherford RB (ed): *Vascular Surgery*, 5th edition. Philadelphia, Saunders, 2000, p 149.

376. A. AC-coupled output.

AC-coupled amplification is appropriate for arterial plethysmography; DC-coupling is appropriate for venous recording.

▷Rumwell CB, McPharlin M: *Vascular Technology: An Illustrated Review*, 5th edition. Pasadena, CA, Davies Publishing, 2015, p 105.

377. C. An absent flow reversal component, blunting of the peak velocity, and prolonged upslope and downslope.

Doppler waveforms distal to a significant stenosis reflect to some degree the loss of energy caused by the stenosis. It has been said that a stenosis acts as a low-pass filter; that is, it tends to filter out the high-frequency changes in the waveform, such as the dicrotic notch.

▷Rumwell CB, McPharlin M: *Vascular Technology: An Illustrated Review*, 5th edition. Pasadena, CA, Davies Publishing, 2015, p 62.

378. A. Changes in thigh-to-ankle index.

Thigh-to-ankle index is not a diagnostic parameter in exercise testing.

▷Zierler RE, Sumner DS: Physiologic assessment of peripheral arterial occlusive disease. In Rutherford RB (ed): *Vascular Surgery*, 5th edition. Philadelphia, Saunders, 2000, p 149.

379. A. Patient's inability to tolerate application of pressure cuffs.

One needs to apply cuffs for both exercise and reactive hyperemia testing. Indeed, some patients cannot tolerate the suprasystolic pressures needed for reactive hyperemia testing.

▷Zierler RE, Sumner DS: Physiologic assessment of peripheral arterial occlusive disease. In Rutherford RB (ed): *Vascular Surgery*, 5th edition. Philadelphia, Saunders, 2000, p 149.

380. E. Reverse-flow component.

The reverse-flow component is part of an arterial Doppler waveform, not a volume waveform, which does not have a zero baseline.

▷Rumwell CB, McPharlin M: *Vascular Technology: An Illustrated Review*, 5th edition. Pasadena, CA, Davies Publishing, 2015, pp 103–105.

381. B. A qualitative approach or pattern recognition.

Most analog Doppler analysis is qualitative—assessing for presence or absence of characteristics, such as the reverse-flow component.

▷Rumwell CB, McPharlin M: *Vascular Technology: An Illustrated Review*, 5th edition. Pasadena, CA, Davies Publishing, 2015, p 62.

382. C. A sharp upslope and downslope and a prominent reverse flow component.

Answer choices A and B are characteristics of venous flow. Answer choice D refers to an abnormal volume recording. Answer choice E is just plain abnormal.

▷Rumwell CB, McPharlin M: *Vascular Technology: An Illustrated Review*, 5th edition. Pasadena, CA, Davies Publishing, 2015, p 62.

383. A. No change.

▷Zwiebel WJ: *Introduction to Vascular Ultrasonography*, 5th edition. Philadelphia, Elsevier Saunders, 2005, p 281.

384. C. Is only marginally meaningful diagnostically.

▷Rumwell CB, McPharlin M: *Vascular Technology: An Illustrated Review*, 5th edition. Pasadena, CA, Davies Publishing, 2015, pp 103–105.

385. E. All of the above.

These errors are less likely using duplex ultrasound.

▷Johnston KW: Processing continuous wave Doppler signals, and analysis of peripheral arterial waveforms: problems and solutions. In Bernstein EF (ed): *Vascular Diagnosis*, 4th edition. St. Louis, Mosby, 1993, p 157.

386. E. A and B only.

Output settings do not affect attenuation; they control size of recording on the chart paper.

▷Johnston KW: Processing continuous wave Doppler signals, and analysis of peripheral arterial waveforms: problems and solutions. In Bernstein EF (ed): *Vascular Diagnosis*, 4th edition. St. Louis, Mosby, 1993, p 157.

387. D. Will appear markedly dampened, possibly making interpretation difficult for distal segments.

Damped waveforms distal to proximal arterial occlusive disease can make the evaluation of further distal disease difficult.

▷Zierler RE, Sumner DS: Physiologic assessment of peripheral arterial occlusive disease. In Rutherford RB (ed): *Vascular Surgery*, 5th edition. Philadelphia, Saunders, 2000, p 153.

388. A. Determination of arterial level of obstruction.

Like ankle/arm indices, $TcPO_2$ can assess only at the site of measurement; it cannot localize the level of proximal obstruction.

▷Rumwell CB, McPharlin M: *Vascular Technology: An Illustrated Review*, 5th edition. Pasadena, CA, Davies Publishing, 2015, p 116.

389. A. 65 mmHg.

▷Zierler RE, Sumner DS: Physiologic assessment of peripheral arterial occlusive disease. In Rutherford RB (ed): *Vascular Surgery*, 5th edition. Philadelphia, Saunders, 2000, p 155.

390. B. Secondary Raynaud's disease.

This finding is not universally supported in the literature.

▷Sumner DS: Mercury strain-gauge plethysmography. In Bernstein EF (ed): *Vascular Diagnosis*, 4th edition. St. Louis, Mosby, 1993, p 218.

391. C. Low-pitched and monophasic.

Any arterial signal distal to a total occlusion represents flow via collaterals; much of the original energy is damped out, although the degree of damping varies with the quality of the collaterals.

▷Rumwell CB, McPharlin M: *Vascular Technology: An Illustrated Review*, 5th edition. Pasadena, CA, Davies Publishing, 2015, p 62.

392. C. May be absent in vasodilated limbs.

Vasodilated limbs have low distal resistance and exhibit the reduction or absence of diastolic flow reversal.

▷Rumwell CB, McPharlin M: *Vascular Technology: An Illustrated Review*, 5th edition. Pasadena, CA, Davies Publishing, 2015, pp 64–65.

393. B. The results are influenced by the patient's peripheral resistance.

Performing the exam in a cold room causes vasoconstriction that may affect peripheral resistance and toe pressures.

▷Carter SA: Role of pressure measurements. In Bernstein EF (ed): *Vascular Diagnosis*, 4th edition. St. Louis, Mosby, 1993, p 490.

394. C. Relatively high-frequency with pulsatile components.

Arterial Doppler signals do not change appreciably with respiration.

▷Pellerito JS, Polak JF: *Introduction to Vascular Ultrasonography*, 6th edition. Philadelphia, Elsevier Saunders, 2012, pp 245–247.

395. D. Have a high-frequency sound.

The accelerated velocities will create high-frequency signals directly in the stenotic jet. Just distally there will be turbulent flow and a scrambled analog waveform—many velocities and many directions causing many frequency shifts, which the analog output cannot deal with.

▷Pellerito JS, Polak JF: *Introduction to Vascular Ultrasonography*, 6th edition. Philadelphia, Elsevier Saunders, 2012, p 246.

396. B. Significant obstructive disease.

A normal PORH response is a major velocity increase; see the next question.

▷Fronek A, Bernstein EF: Postocclusive reactive hyperemia in the testing of the peripheral arterial system: pressure, velocity, and pulse reappearance time. In Bernstein EF (ed): *Vascular Diagnosis*, 4th edition. St. Louis, Mosby, 1993, p 555.

397. A. A > 100% increase in mean velocity.

▷Fronek A, Bernstein EF: Postocclusive reactive hyperemia in the testing of the peripheral arterial system: pressure, velocity, and pulse reappearance time. In Bernstein EF (ed): *Vascular Diagnosis*, 4th edition. St. Louis, Mosby, 1993, p 555.

398. B. The low pass filter may be set too high.

The high pass filter setting on high could clip frequencies near the baseline, leaving only a monophasic waveform above baseline in the normal arterial signal.

▷Ridgway DP: *Introduction to Vascular Scanning*, 4th edition. Pasadena, CA, Davies Publishing, 2014, p 198.

399. A. Less than 0.50.

Actually more likely less than 0.30; this is consistent with ischemic rest pain.

▷Rumwell CB, McPharlin M: *Vascular Technology: An
Illustrated Review*, 5th edition. Pasadena, CA, Davies
Publishing, 2015, pp 46, 75.

400. C. May be in the normal range or abnormally decreased, yet falsely elevated.

Ankle/arm indices in the presence of calcification may indicate the presence of disease or no disease. In either state the pressures may be artificially elevated because of the calcification making the vessels harder to compress. Any pressure taken in a diabetic patient should be analyzed with suspicion.

▷Rumwell CB, McPharlin M: *Vascular Technology: An
Illustrated Review*, 5th edition. Pasadena, CA, Davies
Publishing, 2015, pp 69–70.

401. B. You have stood the probe up, increasing the angle of incidence.

Increasing the angle of incidence would <u>lower</u> the frequency shift. The other items are possible reasons for an <u>increase</u> of frequency shift. The scenario in answer D would decrease the angle, thereby increasing the frequency shift.

▷Rumwell CB, McPharlin M: *Vascular Technology: An
Illustrated Review*, 5th edition. Pasadena, CA, Davies
Publishing, 2015, p 61.

402. D. The graft velocity has dropped from 70 cm/sec, as measured 6 months earlier, to 30 cm/sec.

A graft velocity of 30 cm/sec that has dropped from 70 cm/sec is usually a clear indicator of impending graft failure. It is important to remember that the size of the graft affects flow velocities, and that there may be low velocities within a graft that is especially large or has large-diameter segments, so that velocities of 30 cm/sec by themselves are not necessarily indicative of graft failure.

▷Rumwell CB, McPharlin M: *Vascular Technology: An
Illustrated Review*, 5th edition. Pasadena, CA, Davies
Publishing, 2015, pp 134–136.

403. B. Are falsely elevated less frequently than tibial ankle pressures.

Toe pressures can be a useful adjunct in the diabetic patient with artificially high ankle pressures.

▷Zierler RE, Sumner DS: Physiologic assessment of
peripheral arterial occlusive disease. In Rutherford RB (ed):
Vascular Surgery, 5th edition. Philadelphia, Saunders, 2000, p
146.

404. E. The patient may have aortoiliac occlusive disease.

The patient <u>may</u> have aortoiliac disease (e.g., in the presence of partially calcified femoral artery walls), although without further information about waveforms in the aortoiliac

vessels or at the common femoral level this <u>cannot</u> be precisely determined. "Aortoiliac disease cannot be ruled out" is the phrase often used by readers of pressure studies given this information. Thus, while answer choice A is possible, E is the best (most cautious) assessment of this limited information.

▷Carter SA: Role of pressure measurements. In Bernstein EF
(ed): *Vascular Diagnosis*, 4th edition. St. Louis, Mosby, 1993,
pp 488, 507.

This may seem unnecessarily subtle, but in the exam, as in life, one must constantly be on guard for things waiting to fool you.

405. C. In patients with similar thigh and arm diameters.

Accurate measurement of blood pressure requires a cuff that is 1.2 times the limb diameter. If the arm cuff were 1.2 times the arm and thigh diameter, then it would work for both. The usual situation is use of the four-cuff method, with the high-thigh cuff being narrower than the 1.2 rule for all but the most slender limbs. This almost always leads to some degree of cuff artifact, which we live with in our interpretations.

▷Zwiebel WJ: *Introduction to Vascular Ultrasonography*, 5th
edition. Philadelphia, Elsevier Saunders, 2005, p 278.

▷Rumwell CB, McPharlin M: *Vascular Technology: An
Illustrated Review*, 5th edition. Pasadena, CA, Davies
Publishing, 2015, pp 71, 82.

406. D. Approximately 2 mmHg per heart beat.

Approximately 2 mmHg per heartbeat gives the most accurate measurement of blood pressure; deflating too fast or too slowly may give inaccurate results. It is especially important not to bleed the cuff too quickly for a patient with cardiac arrhythmia.

▷Pellerito JS, Polak JF: *Introduction to Vascular
Ultrasonography*, 6th edition. Philadelphia, Elsevier Saunders,
2012, p 251.

407. B. A double-line appearance of the graft walls.

PTFE (Gore-Tex) graft is characterized by a double-line appearance of the graft walls.

▷Ridgway DA: *Introduction to Vascular Scanning*, 4th edition.
Pasadena, CA, Davies Publishing, 2014, p266–267.

408. E. Will be 100% greater than the prestenotic velocity followed by a drop in velocity.

Absolute velocities will differ depending on the size of graft, but usually a 100% increase in velocity followed by a distal decrease in velocity is indicative of a 50% stenosis.

▷Rumwell CB, McPharlin M: *Vascular Technology: An
Illustrated Review*, 5th edition. Pasadena, CA, Davies
Publishing, 2015, p 135.

409. A. Higher proximally and lower distally.

The velocities will vary depending on the inflow, size of graft, location (and quality) of valve cusps, presence of stenoses, and tightness of distal anastomosis. Generally the velocities in a reversed vein graft will be lower distally (compared to proximal) because of the increased size of the graft distally.

410. C. The same throughout the graft.

The flow rate must be the same throughout the graft, assuming no leaks, even though the velocities may differ: Q = mean V times CSA.

▷Rumwell CB, McPharlin M: *Vascular Technology: An Illustrated Review*, 5th edition. Pasadena, CA, Davies Publishing, 2015, p 23.

411. D. Vasodilatation increases, and distal resistance decreases.

The body attempts to increase nutritive blood flow to the extremity by vasodilatation and the subsequent decrease of peripheral resistance. The drop in distal pressure is a result of the increased segmental resistance and "stealing" of blood to the large muscle groups.

▷Carter SA: Role of pressure measurements. In Bernstein EF (ed): *Vascular Diagnosis*, 4th edition. St. Louis, Mosby, 1993, p 486.

412. B. Proximal to the point of insonation.

This is as specific as you can get with this information. The damped waveform is the result of obstruction damping out energy somewhere proximal to your probe, but you can't yet say exactly where.

413. B. 60–80 mmHg.

▷Rumwell CB, McPharlin M: *Vascular Technology: An Illustrated Review*, 5th edition. Pasadena, CA, Davies Publishing, 2015, p 118.

414. C. Before breakfast.

Patients for AAA or SMA evaluation should be tested first thing in the morning if possible and NPO (nothing by mouth) past midnight to minimize shadowing due to bowel gas.

415. B. Triphasic waveforms at the common femoral and proximal superficial femoral arteries with monophasic waveforms in the popliteal and tibial arteries.

Usually triphasic, but occasionally monophasic, staccato-type waveforms may be seen proximal to an occlusion in the superficial femoral artery.

▷Zierler RE, Sumner DS: Physiologic assessment of
peripheral arterial occlusive disease. In Rutherford RB (ed):
Vascular Surgery, 5th edition. Philadelphia, Saunders, 2000, p
153.

416. A. The higher of the right or left arm pressures.

*It is very important to remember that the higher arm pressure is the pressure used to
determine ankle/brachial systolic pressures.*

▷Rumwell CB, McPharlin M: *Vascular Technology: An
Illustrated Review*, 5th edition. Pasadena, CA, Davies
Publishing, 2015, p 74.

417. C. 1-c and 2-d.

*Claudication usually occurs with indices between 0.50 and 0.80, and rest pain with indices
less than 0.50 (often less than 0.20).*

▷Rumwell CB, McPharlin M: *Vascular Technology: An
Illustrated Review*, 5th edition. Pasadena, CA, Davies
Publishing, 2015, p 75.

418. C. A transient decrease of approximately 20%.

*This decrease is normally quite brief and may not be registered unless pressures are taken
immediately on thigh-cuff deflation.Pellerito says the response may range from 20% to
30%.*

▷Pellerito JS, Polak JF: *Introduction to Vascular
Ultrasonography*, 6th edition. Philadelphia, Elsevier Saunders,
2012, p 256.

419. B. Duplex ultrasonography.

All of the rest of these are able to detect digital pulse and/or changes in arterial volume.

▷Rumwell CB, McPharlin M: *Vascular Technology: An
Illustrated Review*, 5th edition. Pasadena, CA, Davies
Publishing, 2015, pp 99–100.

420. D. Mild iliofemoral stenosis, severe superficial femoral stenosis or occlusion, and severe
infrapopliteal occlusive disease.

*These waveform tracings range from the mildest change (absence of dicrotic notch) to most
severe (flat tracings) as we progress down the leg.*

▷Rumwell CB, McPharlin M: *Vascular Technology: An
Illustrated Review*, 5th edition. Pasadena, CA, Davies
Publishing, 2015, pp 103–105.

421. C. Is vasodilated.

Loss of the dicrotic notch is generally the first abnormality to show in volume recording, but this finding is not definitive. Vasodilatation will often eliminate the dicrotic notch, and since we know nothing about any previous history we cannot state anything about the sympathectomy. Lacunar strokes are unlikely to be related to vasomotor state.

▷Zierler RE, Sumner DS: Physiologic assessment of
peripheral arterial occlusive disease. In Rutherford RB (ed):
Vascular Surgery, 5th edition. Philadelphia, Saunders, 2000, p
155.

422. A. Increase the pulsatility index.

Pulsatility can be informally defined as the degree to which the waveform deviates from the mean. Clenching the fist offers much greater distal resistance, so the Doppler waveform would be expected to become more pulsatile. In addition to increasing the pulsatility index, a closed fist will also decrease the diastolic flow.

▷Rumwell CB, McPharlin M: *Vascular Technology: An
Illustrated Review*, 5th edition. Pasadena, CA, Davies
Publishing, 2015, pp 28–29.

423. A. This statement—"Normal digital pressures when the hand is immersed in cold water"— probably does NOT describe aspects of Raynaud's disease.

Finger pressures after cold water immersion decrease in the patient with Raynaud's secondary to vasoconstriction. Indeed, the pulse usually disappears altogether, making pressure measurement impossible until the spasm passes.

▷Edwards JM, Porter JM: Evaluation of upper extremity
ischemia. In Bernstein EF (ed): *Vascular Diagnosis*, 4th edition.
St. Louis, Mosby, 1993, p 636.

424. B. Coarctation of the aorta.

Both coarctation of the aorta and renal artery stenosis can cause the hypertension, but only coarctation will also cause the abnormal femoral pulses.

425. D. A mask, often without contrast, is selected to be subtracted from the frames obtained during injection of the contrast solution.

Any subtraction technique uses a mask to subtract unnecessary information (such as bony structures) from the final arteriogram.

▷Hodgson KJ: Principles of arteriography. In Rutherford RB
(ed): *Vascular Surgery*, 5th edition. Philadelphia, Saunders,
2000, p 286.

426. D. Patient cooperation.

Patient cooperation is a significant problem with digital subtraction angiography (DSA), as patient motion can drastically affect the ability of DSA to provide adequate images.

▷Hodgson KJ: Principles of arteriography. In Rutherford RB
(ed): *Vascular Surgery*, 5th edition. Philadelphia, Saunders,
2000, p 286.

427. C. This statement about peripheral arterial arteriography—"Arteriography is used for routine postoperative follow-up"—is NOT correct.

Since it is invasive and carries a small but definite risk of complications, arteriography is not used routinely. Adverse reactions are less likely with newer contrast agents, and arteriography is usually performed prior to peripheral arterial surgery.

▷Hodgson KJ: Principles of arteriography. In Rutherford RB
(ed): *Vascular Surgery*, 5th edition. Philadelphia, Saunders,
2000, p 286 ff.

428. B. Common femoral artery.

This is a large, relatively superficial artery that usually provides the easiest access to the arterial system.

▷Rumwell CB, McPharlin M: *Vascular Technology: An
Illustrated Review*, 5th edition. Pasadena, CA, Davies
Publishing, 2015, p 174.

429. D. Aortoiliac, femoropopliteal, and trifurcation arteries.

430. B. Renal failure.

Contrast can cause severe complications in patients with compromised renal function. To be sure, diabetic patients might fall into this category (answer A), but B is the best answer.

▷Hodgson KJ: Principles of arteriography. In Rutherford RB
(ed): *Vascular Surgery*, 5th edition. Philadelphia, Saunders,
2000, p 296.

431. E. Fibromuscular dysplasia.

▷Rumwell CB, McPharlin M: *Vascular Technology: An
Illustrated Review*, 5th edition. Pasadena, CA, Davies
Publishing, 2015, p 177.

432. C. Femoral or popliteal aneurysm.

Answers A, B, and D are possible, but other modalities are more accurate and/or more cost-effective for these problems. Esophageal varices do not occur in the lower extremities.

▷Fillinger MF: Computed tomography and three-dimensional
reconstruction in evaluation of vascular disease. In Rutherford
RB (ed): *Vascular Surgery*, 5th edition. Philadelphia, Saunders,
2000, p 264.

433. A. This statement—"MRA cannot achieve the accuracy of conventional angiography"—is FALSE.

MRA can be as accurate as conventional angiography. The other statements are true.

▷Vlazquez OC, Gaum RA, Carpenter JP: Magnetic resonance imaging and angiography. In Rutherford RB (ed): *Vascular Surgery*, 5th edition. Philadelphia, Saunders, 2000, pp 271–277.

434. B. Worse.

Patency results of femoral and popliteal angioplasty have been consistently poorer than those in the iliac arteries.

▷Schneider PA, Rutherford RB: Endovascular interventions in the management of chronic lower extremity ischemia. In Rutherford RB (ed): *Vascular Surgery*, 5th edition. Philadelphia, Saunders, 2000, p 1055.

435. E. Bifurcations.

This is a method of deploying balloon angioplasty and arranging stents at bifurcations, avoiding occlusion of one branch while dilating the other. The technique can be used anywhere, including coronary arteries.

▷Schneider PA, Rutherford RB: Endovascular interventions in the management of chronic lower extremity ischemia. In Rutherford RB (ed): *Vascular Surgery*, 5th edition. Philadelphia, Saunders, 2000, p 1048.

436. A. In situ saphenous graft.

The valvulatome disables the valves in the unresituated vein, allowing blood to flow unimpeded from proximal to distal. (In situ: in place.)

▷Whittemore AD, Belkin M: Infrainguinal bypass. In Rutherford RB (ed): *Vascular Surgery*, 5th edition. Philadelphia, Saunders, 2000, p 1007.

437. A. Cephalic vein.

The cephalic and basilic veins are the upper extremity veins most commonly used for arterial bypasses. The cephalic vein is used most often.

▷Towne JB: The autogenous vein. In Rutherford RB (ed): *Vascular Surgery*, 5th edition. Philadelphia, Saunders, 2000, p 540.

438. E. The femoral vein.

The femoral vein is not superficial. It is in fact used for autologous vein graft on occasion, however.

This seems as good a time as any to reinforce the necessity to stop using the term "superficial femoral" and simply say "femoral" for the vein running from the deep femoral junction to the adductor hiatus (i.e., between common femoral and popliteal). There are cases of confusion when reporting "femoral vein thrombosis" to referring physicians, who may hear the "superficial" part, consider the thrombosis less than urgent, and just send the patient home. Therefore, using just "femoral" makes sense, at least for reporting purposes. (The artery can still be "superficial femoral artery," however.) This change in nomenclature, along with the establishment of "great saphenous" and "small saphenous" as the proper terms for those veins, was mandated by an international group of venous luminaries, so we should get with it.

▷Towne JB: The autogenous vein. In Rutherford RB (ed):
Vascular Surgery, 5th edition. Philadelphia, Saunders, 2000, p
540.

439. B. This statement—"The risk of death from cardiac disease is greater than the risk of death from rupture of the aneurysm"—is FALSE.

Despite the association of cardiac disease with other manifestations of atherosclerosis, patients with unrepaired aneurysms of this size have a higher mortality due to rupture than to cardiac disease. Despite the size, the occurrence of other complications is not that common. Before the advent of elective surgical repair, patients with aneurysms were followed extensively in some series, so the natural history of the disease is well known. Most patients choose surgery to reduce their risk of death related to rupture.

▷Cronenwett JL, Krupski WC, Rutherford RB: Abdominal aortic
and iliac aneurysms. In Rutherford RB (ed): *Vascular Surgery*,
5th edition. Philadelphia, Saunders, 2000, p 1253.

440. A. Femorofemoral bypass.

Since this patient's left iliac artery is totally occluded, there is no indication for femoropopliteal bypass, lumbar sympathectomy, or balloon angioplasty. Although axillofemoral bypass is a viable alternative, it is seldom performed in preference to the femorofemoral bypass, which is the procedure of choice for this patient.

▷Rutherford RB: Extra-anatomic bypass. In Rutherford RB
(ed): *Vascular Surgery*, 5th edition. Philadelphia, Saunders,
2000, p 984.

441. E. <10%.

There is a very small risk of rupture with a 4 cm aneurysm; the risk increases to 3–15% per year at 5–6 cm, and 30–50% per year at 8 cm or larger. Other risk factors figure into the risk of rupture.

▷Cronenwett JL, Krupski WC, Rutherford RB: Abdominal aortic
and iliac aneurysms. In Rutherford RB (ed): *Vascular Surgery*,
5th edition. Philadelphia, Saunders, 2000, p 1255.

442. D. Potentially useful in claudicating patients.

Sympathectomy is unlikely to be useful in claudicators.

▷Rutherford RB: Lumbar sympathectomy: indications and technique. In Rutherford RB (ed): *Vascular Surgery*, 5th edition. Philadelphia, Saunders, 2000, p 1072.

443. A. tPA.

The usual thrombolytic of choice is tPA (tissue plasminogen activator).

444. A. Elective repair.

The risk of rupture increases dramatically as an abdominal aortic aneurysm exceeds 5 to 6 cm in diameter.

▷Pellerito JS, Polak JF: *Introduction to Vascular Ultrasonography*, 6th edition. Philadelphia, Elsevier Saunders, 2012, pp 454–455.

ABDOMINAL & VISCERAL VASCULAR DISEASE

445. C. Renal/aortic ratio.

Renovascular hypertension is caused by renal artery stenosis. Stenosis of the renal artery can be determined by obtaining a renal/aortic ratio (RAR). This is a ratio of the highest velocity obtained in the renal artery to the normal velocity of the aorta obtained at the level of the renal artery origins. A ratio of ≥ 3.5 is considered by most to indicate a significant renal artery stenosis. This would mean that the velocity in the renal artery is 3.5 times faster than the velocity in the aorta.

▷Rumwell CB, McPharlin M: *Vascular Technology: An Illustrated Review*, 5th edition. Pasadena, CA, Davies Publishing, 2015, p 145.

446. D. Celiac artery.

The median arcuate ligament of the diaphragm crosses the anterior aspect of the aorta slightly above (i.e., superior to) the celiac trunk. In some patients, during expiration, this anatomic situation can lead to compression of the celiac artery and high velocities. The abnormally high velocities are present during expiration but return to normal during inspiration. These patients may present with an abdominal bruit.

▷Rumwell CB, McPharlin M: *Vascular Technology: An Illustrated Review*, 5th edition. Pasadena, CA, Davies Publishing, 2015, p 153.

447. A. Proximal.

Atherosclerotic disease tends to affect the bifurcations of arteries. The renal artery is most commonly affected at its origin from the aorta. This is considered to be the proximal portion of the vessel. Fibromuscular disease more commonly affects the mid to distal aspect of the renal artery.

448. C. Decreased flow resistance in parenchymal arteries is NOT a common feature of renal allograft rejection.

In renal allograft rejection the flow resistance in the parenchymal arteries tends to increase. This will be manifested as a decrease in diastolic flow. Normal flow in the parenchymal arteries of a renal allograft is low-resistance with forward flow throughout the cardiac cycle. A decrease, absence, or reversal of flow in diastole is indicative of rejection.

▷Rumwell CB, McPharlin M: *Vascular Technology: An Illustrated Review*, 5th edition. Pasadena, CA, Davies Publishing, 2015, pp 155–157.

449. D. Enlarged coronary vein.

The coronary vein normally drains into the splenic vein. With portal hypertension, the increased portal venous pressure decreases flow into the portal system. Consequently, vessels that normally drain into the portal system become enlarged and often find alternate routes of flow. The coronary vein may reverse its flow direction and feed into esophageal varices. These can break down, causing life-threatening bleeding episodes. Cavernous transformation may occur in patients with portal hypertension, but only in the presence of portal vein thrombosis and recanalization. Cavernous transformation of the portal vein most commonly occurs when the liver is normal. Most patients with portal hypertension have underlying liver cirrhosis. Aortic dissection and hepatic artery aneurysm are not associated with portal hypertension.

450. B. Portal hypertension.

This is one of several possible collateral pathways through which flow from the intestine reaches the inferior vena cava in the event of abnormally increased portal vein resistance (i.e., cirrhosis).

▷Pellerito JS, Polak JF: *Introduction to Vascular Ultrasonography*, 6th edition. Philadelphia, Elsevier Saunders, 2012, pp 497–504.

451. D. Hepatic vein obstruction.

Hepatic vein obstruction leaves no way for portal venous hepatic arterial blood to be removed. Therefore hepatic congestion occurs, resulting in ascites, progressive hepatic dysfunction, and portal hypertension. In its acute form the disease is rapidly fatal, unless treated surgically. Liver tumors are a separate possible cause of hepatic vein obstruction.

▷Johansen KH, Helton WS, Rikkers LF: Operative therapy for portal hypertension. In Rutherford RB (ed): *Vascular Surgery*, 5th edition. Philadelphia, Saunders, 2000, p 1578.

452. B. Cirrhosis.

453. A. Celiac artery, superior mesenteric artery, inferior mesenteric artery.

The splanchnic arteries are the vessels that supply blood to the gut. These primarily are the celiac artery, superior mesenteric artery (SMA), and inferior mesenteric artery (IMA). Stenosis or occlusion involving these vessels can result in chronic ischemia of the bowel, known as mesenteric ischemia.

454. B. Malnourished.

Since eating causes severe ischemic abdominal pain, patients with mesenteric ischemia tend to avoid eating and to have pronounced weight loss.

▷Pellerito JS, Polak JF: *Introduction to Vascular Ultrasonography*, 6th edition. Philadelphia, Elsevier Saunders, 2012, p 483.

455. C. Postprandial pain.

This is sometimes referred to as "bowel claudication," since it is ischemic pain brought on by increased demand for perfusion.

▷Pellerito JS, Polak JF: *Introduction to Vascular Ultrasonography*, 6th edition. Philadelphia, Elsevier Saunders, 2012, p 483.

456. E. Claudication.

The others are all possible manifestations of hepatic dysfunction.

▷Johansen KH: Portal hypertension: an overview. In Rutherford RB (ed): *Vascular Surgery*, 5th edition. Philadelphia, Saunders, 2000, p 1550–1551.

457. C. Bleeding esophageal varices.

This results from abnormally high venous pressures due to cirrhosis or other liver disorders. As noted elsewhere, esophageal hemorrhage is often lethal.

▷Johansen KH: Portal hypertension: an overview. In
Rutherford RB (ed): *Vascular Surgery*, 5th edition.
Philadelphia, Saunders, 2000, p 1550–1551.

458. C. Superior mesenteric artery.

Chronic mesenteric ischemia may result from obstruction of the arteries that supply the gut. The primary vessel supplying the intestine is the superior mesenteric artery. The inferior mesenteric artery and celiac trunk may also contribute. Symptoms usually do not occur unless 2 of these 3 arteries are obstructed. A rich collateral network exists between these three vessels, making chronic mesenteric ischemia a rare disorder.

▷Baxter BT, Pearce WH: Diagnosis and surgical management
of chronic mesenteric ischemia. In Strandness DE, van Breda
A (eds): *Vascular Diseases: Surgical and Interventional
Therapy*. New York, Churchill Livingstone, 1994, pp 795–802.

459. D. Portal hypertension.

460. C. Requires a duplex system with spectral signal analysis.

Low-frequency ultrasound probes can image structures in the retroperitoneal space, but their images are not of sufficient quality to demonstrate plaque; the only studies utilized for this type of assessment have been with a Doppler. However, an imaging system is critical to assure that the correct vessel is being sampled.

▷Burns PN: Principles of deep Doppler ultrasonography. In
Bernstein EF (ed): *Vascular Diagnosis*, 4th edition. St. Louis,
Mosby, 1993, p 249.

461. E. Superior mesenteric.

After eating (i.e., postprandially), vasodilatation in the intestine reduces distal resistance.

▷Rumwell CB, McPharlin M: *Vascular Technology: An
Illustrated Review*, 5th edition. Pasadena, CA, Davies
Publishing, 2015, pp 150–151.

462. C. Are low-resistance in character (much diastolic flow).

▷Pellerito JS, Polak JF: *Introduction to Vascular
Ultrasonography*, 6th edition. Philadelphia, Elsevier Saunders,
2012, pp 519–521.

463. D. Systolic renal/aortic velocity ratio is greater than 3.5.

Renal to aortic ratios that are > 3.5 are a common method of detecting proximal renal artery stenosis. Another method, which requires the localization of the stenosis, is to see a velocity increase of 100% or more from the prestenotic velocity.

▷Rumwell CB, McPharlin M: *Vascular Technology: An
Illustrated Review*, 5th edition. Pasadena, CA, Davies
Publishing, 2015, p 145.

464. B. Superior and inferior mesenteric artery.

In order for there to be intestinal ischemia, severe stenoses must be present in two of the three main supplying arteries (celiac, superior mesenteric, and inferior mesenteric).

▷Pellerito JS, Polak JF: *Introduction to Vascular Ultrasonography*, 6th edition. Philadelphia, Elsevier Saunders, 2012, pp 480–482.

465. E. Renal stenosis/aorta peak systolic velocity ratio greater than 3.5.

Renal to aortic ratios of greater than 3.5 are associated with renal artery stenosis of greater than 60%.

▷Rumwell CB, McPharlin M: *Vascular Technology: An Illustrated Review*, 5th edition. Pasadena, CA, Davies Publishing, 2015, p 145.

466. A. Augment.

467. B. Portal hypertension.

Portal vein flow is normally gently phasic with respiration and not pulsatile in character.

▷Pellerito JS, Polak JF: *Introduction to Vascular Ultrasonography*, 6th edition. Philadelphia, Elsevier Saunders, 2012, pp 498–499.

468. A. Normally is phasic with respiration.

▷Pellerito JS, Polak JF: *Introduction to Vascular Ultrasonography*, 6th edition. Philadelphia, Elsevier Saunders, 2012, p 498.

469. C. Bidirectional.

This is the result of this vessel's proximity to the right atrium; it reflects right atrial pressure changes.

▷Pellerito JS, Polak JF: *Introduction to Vascular Ultrasonography*, 6th edition. Philadelphia, Elsevier Saunders, 2012, p 495.

470. C. The patient taking a quick, deep breath.

Because it is usually difficult to perform compression maneuvers at this level, this big sniff is a useful way to assess at the subclavian level.

▷Talbot SR: Venous imaging technique. In Talbot SR, Oliver MA: *Techniques of Venous Imaging.* Pasadena, CA, Davies Publishing, 1992, p 105.

471. B. Pulsatile.

The presence of pulsatility, reflecting right atrial activity, should be noted. Its absence may suggest obstruction between the right atrium and the subclavian vein.

▷Pellerito JS, Polak JF: *Introduction to Vascular Ultrasonography*, 6th edition. Philadelphia, Elsevier Saunders, 2012, pp 371–372.

472. D. Bidirectional.

Due to the proximity to the right atrium, hepatic vein flow is normally bidirectional and reflects right-atrial pressure changes.

▷Pellerito JS, Polak JF: *Introduction to Vascular Ultrasonography*, 6th edition. Philadelphia, Elsevier Saunders, 2012, p 495.

473. C. Hepatic vein.

This condition results from acute obstruction of the hepatic vein.

▷Pellerito JS, Polak JF: *Introduction to Vascular Ultrasonography*, 6th edition. Philadelphia, Elsevier Saunders, 2012, p 510.

474. B. Hepatopetal flow in the main portal vein.

Flow should be hepatopetal: toward the liver. Hepatofugal flow, away from the liver, is an abnormal finding in both the portal and splenic veins. No flow is bad too.

▷Pellerito JS, Polak JF: *Introduction to Vascular Ultrasonography*, 6th edition. Philadelphia, Elsevier Saunders, 2012, p 512.

475. A. Cirrhosis.

The most common cause of portal hypertension in the industrialized western world is cirrhosis. (Elsewhere, hepatitis is the usual cause.) The TIPS helps to relieve the excess pressure.

▷Pellerito JS, Polak JF: *Introduction to Vascular Ultrasonography*, 6th edition. Philadelphia, Elsevier Saunders, 2012, p 497.

MISCELLANEOUS CONDITIONS & TESTS

476. A. Use color flow to confirm that flow remains biphasic within the pseudoaneurysm.

Ultrasound-guided thrombin injection looks promising at press time and may eventually replace this strenuous procedure.

▷Pellerito JS, Polak JF: *Introduction to Vascular Ultrasonography*, 6th edition. Philadelphia, Elsevier Saunders, 2012, pp 331–334.

477. A. Increasing.

As the number of transluminal procedures increases, we are seeing more iatrogenic pseudoaneurysms.

▷Schwartz LB, Clark ET, Gewertz BL: Anastomotic and other pseudoaneurysms. In Rutherford RB (ed): *Vascular Surgery*, 5th edition. Philadelphia, Saunders, 2000, p 753.

478. B. Penile pressure can decrease after treadmill testing.

Vascular disease is the most common cause of impotence, but neurogenic and psychosomatic causes are also possible. Penile pressures can decrease after exercise as a result of a steal to the legs when the lower extremity vascular resistance is reduced. Any vascular lesion at or above the internal iliac artery may be implicated. Often an erection can be initiated but not sustained. Surgical correction of the vascular disease is at this time done only in selected cases, with promising but not absolute results.

▷Zwiebel WJ: *Introduction to Vascular Ultrasonography*, 5th edition. Philadelphia, Elsevier Saunders, 2005, p 673.

▷DePalma RG, Kempczinski RF: Vasculogenic impotence. In Rutherford RB (ed): *Vascular Surgery*, 5th edition. Philadelphia, Saunders, 2000, p 1102 ff.

479. E. The vein might be used because the graft diameter is 2 mm and might expand under pressure.

Depending on the institution, 2 mm veins might be used as grafts, although the surgeon would likely prefer 3 mm or larger. Duplex measurements taken with just intravenous pressure may not predict the potential diameter with arterial pressure.

▷Towne JB: The autogenous vein. In Rutherford RB (ed): *Vascular Surgery*, 5th edition. Philadelphia, Saunders, 2000, p 545.

▷Kupinski AM, Leather RP, Chang BB, et al: Preoperative mapping of the saphenous vein. In Bernstein EF (ed): *Vascular Diagnosis*, 4th edition. St. Louis, Mosby, 1993, p 901.

480. C. Lack of diastolic flow is abnormal for the transplanted kidney.

Absence of diastolic flow in the transplanted kidney suggests rejection. Other causes of failure, such as ischemic cytosporine injury, may be shown by increased resistance.

▷Pellerito JS, Polak JF: *Introduction to Vascular Ultrasonography*, 6th edition. Philadelphia, Elsevier Saunders, 2012, pp 581–583.

481. E. > 0.75.

Normal penile/brachial index is expressed as greater than 0.75 at rest and not decreasing by more than 0.15 after exercise.

▷Rumwell CB, McPharlin M: *Vascular Technology: An Illustrated Review*, 5th edition. Pasadena, CA, Davies Publishing, 2015, p 95.

482. C. Arteriovenous fistula.

The abrupt change of flow character, and the high diastolic flow in the proximal segment, suggest an AV fistula creating a localized low-resistance pathway.

▷Rumwell CB, McPharlin M: *Vascular Technology: An Illustrated Review*, 5th edition. Pasadena, CA, Davies Publishing, 2015, p 165.

483. A. Saphenous vein mapping prior to bypass surgery.

This frequency is best for fairly superficial structures; it would be too high a frequency for routine lower extremity deep vein assessment.

▷Talbot SR: Venous imaging technique. In Talbot SR, Oliver MA: *Techniques of Venous Imaging*. Pasadena, CA, Davies Publishing, 1992, p 60.

484. E. Less than 200 ml/min.

A flow rate of around 300 ml/min is required for dialysis.

▷Pellerito JS, Polak JF: *Introduction to Vascular Ultrasonography*, 6th edition. Philadelphia, Elsevier Saunders, 2012, pp 287–289.

485. E. Cimino-Brescia.

The flow rates in this type of dialysis fistula are expected to be somewhat lower than those in a PTFE (synthetic) graft.

▷Zwiebel WJ: *Introduction to Vascular Ultrasonography*, 5th edition. Philadelphia, Elsevier Saunders, 2005, p 328.

▷Ridgway DP: *Introduction to Vascular Scanning*, 4th edition. Pasadena, CA, Davies Publishing, 2014, pp 300–301.

486. E. Should not be measured.

One avoids taking brachial blood pressure in an extremity with a dialysis fistula. (Ask any nurse.) You could measure the contralateral brachial blood pressure, of course.

487. C. High, pulsatile venous flow in the veins proximal to the fistula.

The four components of an AV fistula are proximal artery, distal artery, proximal vein, distal vein—and then of course there is the fistula itself. Flow in the proximal artery becomes low-resistance in character (lots of diastolic flow), since the fistula and vein offer much less resistance than the usual vascular bed. Flow in the proximal vein increases and becomes somewhat pulsatile because of the direct arterial inflow and higher volume.

▷Rumwell CB, McPharlin M: *Vascular Technology: An Illustrated Review*, 5th edition. Pasadena, CA, Davies Publishing, 2015, p 165.

488. A. Reduced.

There will be less pressure distally due to the steal across the fistula. All of these flow changes will vary with the size of the fistula, proximity to the heart, and time.

▷Rumwell CB, McPharlin M: *Vascular Technology: An Illustrated Review*, 5th edition. Pasadena, CA, Davies Publishing, 2015, p 166.

489. D. A multitude of arteriovenous channels.

A congenital fistula (AV malformation) usually has many small channels from artery to vein. An acquired (traumatic or dialysis) fistula has a single channel.

▷Rutherford RB, Sumner DS: Diagnostic evaluation of arteriovenous fistulae. In Rutherford RB (ed): *Vascular Surgery*, 5th edition. Philadelphia, Saunders, 2000, p 1432.

490. A. High flow rates exceeding 300 ml/min.

The fistula should have fairly high flow rates to allow for dialysis. The other answer choices are possible abnormalities to look for when scanning.

▷Zwiebel WJ: *Introduction to Vascular Ultrasonography*, 5th edition. Philadelphia, Elsevier Saunders, 2005, pp 334–336.

▷Ridgway DP: *Introduction to Vascular Scanning*, 4th edition. Pasadena, CA, Davies Publishing, 2014, p 301.

491. C. Nerve and/or motor dysfunction due to compartment syndrome may occur without any alteration of arterial hemodynamics.

The anterior tibial artery is located in the anterior compartment and supplies the dorsalis pedis artery. However, increased pressures that can affect anterior tibial nerve and muscle function may be less than those that alter the pressure or audible Doppler characteristics of the anterior tibial artery. The diagnosis of compartment syndrome is made clinically, and, if necessary, intracompartment pressures are measured by a needle/manometer technique.

▷Johansen KH, Watson JC: Compartment syndrome: pathophysiology, recognition, and management. In Rutherford

RB (ed): *Vascular Surgery*, 5th edition. Philadelphia, Saunders, 2000, p 904.

492. C. Thoracic outlet syndrome.

▷Rumwell CB, McPharlin M: *Vascular Technology: An Illustrated Review*, 5th edition. Pasadena, CA, Davies Publishing, 2015, p 170.

493. C. Hobbs maneuver.

The other answer choices are maneuvers that may produce diminished or absent distal arterial flow as monitored by PPG, Doppler, etc. Unfortunately, these results may be obtained in many people without symptoms as well.

▷Rumwell CB, McPharlin M: *Vascular Technology: An Illustrated Review*, 5th edition. Pasadena, CA, Davies Publishing, 2015, p 171.

494. B. Subclavian artery.

495. C. Intimal thickening.

Temporal arteritis causes marked thickening of the intima. It may be localized, focal, or widespread. Patients tend to present with severe headache. Other symptoms may include scalp tenderness, visual disturbance, joint pain, and painful chewing. Blindness can occur as a result of ischemic optic neuropathy in fewer than 20% of patients.

▷Beers MH, Berkow R (eds): *The Merck Manual*, 17th ed. Whitehouse Station, NJ, Merck.

496. C. Several centimeters proximal to the hepatic hilum.

▷Foley WD: *Color Doppler Flow Imaging.* Boston, Andover Medical Publishers, 1991.

497. A. Cephalic vein.

The lesser saphenous, cephalic, and/or basilic veins may be mapped as possible conduits for bypass surgery when the saphenous vein is too small, diseased, or absent. Deep veins such as the deep femoral, popliteal, or axillary are not used.

498. D. Use a high-frequency probe and light probe pressure to track the saphenous vein.

The highest-frequency linear array probe available should be used to track the saphenous vein because it is very superficial. Very light probe pressure should be used since it is easy to compress the vein by resting the probe on the skin. When the vein cannot be visualized, decreasing probe pressure will often help to demonstrate the vein. If the room temperature is too cold, the veins will be small and hard to see. The patient should be placed in a supine position with the leg externally rotated and the knee slightly bent.

▷Talbot SR: Venous imaging technique. In Talbot SR, Oliver MA: *Techniques of Venous Imaging.* Pasadena, Davies Publishing, 1992, pp 59–118.

QUALITY ASSURANCE

499. D. Positive predictive value.

The positive predictive value (PPV) of an examination is the ability of a test to predict the presence of disease (i.e., to predict that the gold standard test will be positive). A positive predictive value of 83% means that you can be 83% sure a positive examination indicates the presence of disease in a given patient.

▷Rumwell CB, McPharlin M: *Vascular Technology: An Illustrated Review,* 5th edition. Pasadena, CA, Davies Publishing, 2015, pp 355–362.

500. B. The positive predictive value will increase, the negative predictive value will decrease, and the accuracy may increase or decrease.

This increase of the threshold raises the bar, as it were, and means that more of the patients called positive by duplex do indeed have severe stenosis. This means an increase in false negatives, since you have increased the PSV required to call severe stenosis. The benefit would be making quite sure that someone designated positive—and perhaps going to surgery—really is positive.

▷Rumwell CB, McPharlin M: *Vascular Technology: An Illustrated Review,* 5th edition. Pasadena, CA, Davies Publishing, 2015, pp 355–362.

501. C. 85%.

Overall accuracy must fall between sensitivity and specificity and between positive predictive and negative predictive values. Answer choice C is the only response that meets these criteria.

▷Rumwell CB, McPharlin M: *Vascular Technology: An Illustrated Review,* 5th edition. Pasadena, CA, Davies Publishing, 2015, pp 355–362.

502. C. 375/400.

For these questions, start by making a 2 x 2 table like the one on the following page:

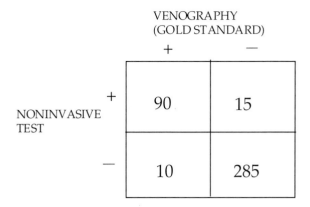

VENOGRAPHY
(GOLD STANDARD)

NONINVASIVE TEST	+	−
+	90	15
−	10	285

Of 400 total exams, 90 were true positives and 285 were true negatives. Accuracy equals all the agreements (positive and negative) divided by all the tests.

▷Rumwell CB, McPharlin M: *Vascular Technology: An Illustrated Review*, 5th edition. Pasadena, CA, Davies Publishing, 2015, pp 355–362.

503. E. 90/100.

Of 100 abnormal venograms, 90 were true positives. Sensitivity equals the positive agreements divided by all of the gold standard positives.

▷Rumwell CB, McPharlin M: *Vascular Technology: An Illustrated Review*, 5th edition. Pasadena, CA, Davies Publishing, 2015, pp 355–362.

504. A. 90/105.

Of 105 abnormal noninvasive exams, 90 were true positives. Positive predictive value equals the positive agreements divided by all of the noninvasive positives.

▷Rumwell CB, McPharlin M: *Vascular Technology: An Illustrated Review*, 5th edition. Pasadena, CA, Davies Publishing, 2015, pp 355–362.

505. E. Negative predictive value.

Overall accuracy has as its denominator the total number of tests performed (all four boxes in the 2 x 2 table).

Specificity has as its denominator the total number of normal (negative) gold-standard studies (i.e., true negatives + false positives, a sum that always equals the number of negative gold-standard results).

Sensitivity has as its denominator the total number of abnormal (positive) gold-standard studies (i.e., true positives + false negatives, a sum that always equals the number of positive gold standard results).

The <u>positive predictive value</u> has as its denominator the total number of abnormal (positive) noninvasive studies, whether true or not (i.e., true positives + false positives).

And finally, <u>negative predictive value</u> has as its denominator the total number of negative noninvasive studies (true negatives + false negatives).

▷Rumwell CB, McPharlin M: *Vascular Technology: An Illustrated Review*, 5th edition. Pasadena, CA, Davies Publishing, 2015, pp 355–362.

506. C. 92.3%.

Again, accuracy must fall between sensitivity and specificity.

▷Rumwell CB, McPharlin M: *Vascular Technology: An Illustrated Review*, 5th edition. Pasadena, CA, Davies Publishing, 2015, pp 355–362.

507. A. 53/61.

As noted above, the denominator for positive predictive value is all the positive noninvasive tests (both true positive and false positive). The numerator is simply the agreements as to positive—you said positive, angio said positive. Note the relationship in the following 2 x 2 table:

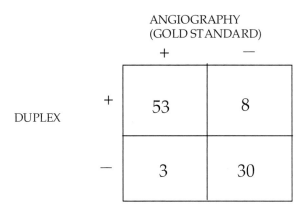

ANGIOGRAPHY
(GOLD STANDARD)

	+	−
DUPLEX +	53	8
−	3	30

▷Rumwell CB, McPharlin M: *Vascular Technology: An Illustrated Review*, 5th edition. Pasadena, CA, Davies Publishing, 2015, pp 355–362.

508. D. 30/38.

The specificity of a test is defined as its ability to exclude disease and to detect normality, expressed as a percentage (the number of true negative tests divided by the total number of negative gold-standard tests, i.e., the true negatives + false positives). In this problem, 38 ICAs had less than 60% stenosis by angiography; this number becomes the denominator in the equation. Thus the numerator is the number correctly classified as normal by the

noninvasive test (i.e., the true negatives, the agreements), in this case 30. Therefore answer choice D is correct.

▷Rumwell CB, McPharlin M: *Vascular Technology: An Illustrated Review*, 5th edition. Pasadena, CA, Davies Publishing, 2015, pp 355–362.

509. E. The negative predictive value is greater than the positive predictive value.

Answer choices A and B can be rejected immediately, since the overall accuracy must fall between the sensitivity and specificity as well as between the positive and negative predictive values. Thus accuracy can be neither lower nor higher than either of the companion measures. Rough calculations can be quickly made for those pertinent measures:

Sensitivity = 53/56 (~90%)
Positive predictive value = 53/61 (~85%)
Specificity = 30/38 (~70%)
Negative predictive value = 30/33 (~91%)

After making these rough calculations, you can reject answer choices C and D and accept answer choice E.

▷Rumwell CB, McPharlin M: *Vascular Technology: An Illustrated Review*, 5th edition. Pasadena, CA, Davies Publishing, 2015, pp 355–362.

510. C. Upper right box.

The mainstream arrangement of the 2 x 2 table looks like this:

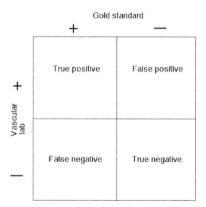

True positives (they say positive, you say positive) go in the upper left box.
True negatives (they say negative, you say negative) go in the lower right box.
False negatives (you say negative, but they say positive) go in the lower left box.
False positives (you say positive, but they say negative) go in the upper right box.

▷Rumwell CB, McPharlin M: *Vascular Technology: An Illustrated Review*, 5th edition. Pasadena, CA, Davies Publishing, 2015, pp 355–362.

511. E. Overall accuracy is calculated by the formula 90/100.

The overall accuracy is the number of correctly classified test results divided by the total number of tests. In this example there are 180 correct test results in the 200 tests performed; thus the correct calculation for overall accuracy is 180/200. The remaining measurements in this problem happen all to be calculated by the formula 90/100.

▷Rumwell CB, McPharlin M: *Vascular Technology: An Illustrated Review*, 5th edition. Pasadena, CA, Davies Publishing, 2015, pp 355–362.

512. C. Of all positive noninvasive tests, 86% correctly predicted that the gold standard would be abnormal.

The calculation of the positive predictive value utilizes only those tests with an abnormal result. Thus any response that utilizes all tests—i.e., responses A and D—cannot be correct. In addition, answer choice B is the definition of sensitivity, since the abnormal "gold standard" results are the denominator of the equation. Thus only responses C and E are potentially correct. Response E states that 14 positive tests were incorrect; this would be true only if a total of 100 positive tests were performed. Since the problem does not state the number of tests performed, there is insufficient data present to derive this answer, and it must be false. The correct definition for the positive value is expressed in response C.

▷Rumwell CB, McPharlin M: *Vascular Technology: An Illustrated Review*, 5th edition. Pasadena, CA, Davies Publishing, 2015, pp 355–362.

513. E. It must be a value from 0 to 100%.

The sensitivity and specificity are mathematically unrelated. The two calculations utilize all the data points in the series, but no single data point is used in both; that is, the two groups are mutually exclusive. Thus, for a value of sensitivity, the specificity can be any value.

▷Rumwell CB, McPharlin M: *Vascular Technology: An Illustrated Review*, 5th edition. Pasadena, CA, Davies Publishing, 2015, pp 355–362.

514. D. The denominator for calculating positive predictive value is 18.

In this example the "gold standard" is not a test, but an outcome: the healing of the amputation site. This time, "abnormal" in the gold standard means not healing, and "abnormal" in the noninvasive test means < 60 mmHg ankle pressure. This can be confusing: It is important to keep clear what is designated "normal" and "abnormal," positive vs. negative. "Positive" here means < 60 mmHg/not healing. Looking at the 2 x 2 table, the denominators for the sensitivity and specificity calculations are the <u>column</u>

totals, not the row totals. The denominator for overall accuracy is the total number of studies, not the total number of correct studies. The predictive values will derive the denominator from the row totals. Thus only answer choice D is correct.

▷Rumwell CB, McPharlin M: *Vascular Technology: An Illustrated Review*, 5th edition. Pasadena, CA, Davies Publishing, 2015, pp 355–362.

515. D. 15/18.

Positive predictive value is calculated by dividing the true positives (agreements) by all of the noninvasive positives (including the false positives).

▷Rumwell CB, McPharlin M: *Vascular Technology: An Illustrated Review*, 5th edition. Pasadena, CA, Davies Publishing, 2015, pp 355–362.

516. C. This statement—"Diabetics with > 60 mmHg ankle pressures that did not heal had calcific arteries causing falsely elevated pressure"— is NOT true based on the data presented.

Ten of 22 diabetics and 10 of 32 nondiabetics did not heal at the amputation site (so A is true). In both groups a pressure of > 60 mmHg was a better indicator of healing potential (so B is true). About 1/3 of patients in both groups had pressures < 60 mmHg; these data do not answer the question of whether calcification of arteries in diabetics elevates the pressure (so D is true). Three of 18 patients with < 60 mmHg did heal at the amputation site (so E is true). Although answer choice C is quite possible, it cannot be verified from this information and is therefore not true.

▷Rumwell CB, McPharlin M: *Vascular Technology: An Illustrated Review*, 5th edition. Pasadena, CA, Davies Publishing, 2015, pp 355–362.

517. A. Zero.

A Kappa value of zero indicates that the observed results occurred because of chance— absolutely no relationship. A Kappa of 1.0 indicates complete agreement between the two variables.

518. D. Call a code.

The very first thing to do is to get the emergency team on its way, since any measures you are capable of taking are strictly temporary. Call 911 if the incident occurs in a facility that does not have a code team or other procedure. Many labs and institutions have written policies and procedures that cover medical and other emergencies. Familiarize yourself with the emergency procedures and follow them when the need arises.

519. D. Guide the fall, protecting his head.

You shouldn't try to arrest the fall, since that may simply injure both of you. The main thing to try is to protect the patient's head, guiding the fall if possible.

HALL OF IMAGES

520. D. Acoustic shadowing.

This is a heavily calcified plaque that creates acoustic shadowing. Calling ulceration with duplex is dodgy in the best of circumstances, and this is not one of those times.

521. C. It suggests severe velocity increase, compatible with approximately 75% stenosis.

Peak systolic velocities this high are compatible with high-grade arterial stenosis. Note the absence of systolic window and some low velocities showing below the baseline, both suggesting pronounced turbulence.

522. D. They suggest aortic valve regurgitation.

The flow during diastole is being pulled retrograde by the aortic valve regurgitation. This isn't seen in the ICA because of the lower-resistance character of the distal vascular bed, but there is the abnormal double peak.

523. E. They suggest graft infection.

The huge area of fluid accumulation around the graft is characteristic of graft infection. Note the double-wall echo created by the graft. This appearance is characteristic of Gore-Tex material.

524. B. It suggests transitional vertebral steal.

Flow is pulled retrograde during systole, then reverts to antegrade during diastole. This suggests a changing abnormal pressure gradient caused by the progression of proximal subclavian artery obstruction.

525. C. Lower on the left.

You would expect lower pressure on the left due to the left subclavian obstruction.

526. A. The exercise causes flow to become retrograde throughout the cardiac cycle.

The exercise increases the demand in the arm, increasing the abnormal pressure gradient and causing flow in the vertebral artery to flow retrograde throughout the cardiac cycle. The patient will not necessarily suffer any symptoms at all.

527. D. Borderline for 80% stenosis.

The end-diastolic velocity is around the borderline for calling a stenosis greater than 80% by most criteria. EDV would not be especially accelerated in a 50% stenosis, and would be expected to be a good deal higher for the designation ">90% stenosis" (kind of a figure of speech meant to convey really, really severe rather than an attempt to be especially accurate).

528. B. Acute venous thrombosis.

This is an acute-appearing venous thrombus: The echoes are very soft and homogeneous, and the thrombus does not appear to adhere very well to the wall. Chronic thrombus would tend to appear brighter and more heterogeneous.

529. A. It suggests turbulent flow.

The shredded appearance and the filling in of the systolic window suggest turbulent flow. There are also some low velocities at systole beneath the baseline. Since turbulent flow goes many directions, mostly at lower velocities, many frequency shifts (some below baseline) are created.

530. E. C and D.

Once again, peak systolic velocities of 500 cm/sec suggest high-grade stenosis; this again looks turbulent.

531. C. Homogeneous plaque that appears to create moderate (<50% stenosis).

This plaque is homogeneous in character; heterogeneous plaque would have mixed soft and bright echoes. It looks like a 40–50% stenosis in this view, certainly not >80%, but estimating stenosis in the longitudinal view can be dangerous.

▷Pellerito JS, Polak JF: *Introduction to Vascular Ultrasonography*, 6th edition. Philadelphia, Elsevier Saunders, 2012, pp 149–151.

532. E. Lymph node.

This is a lymph node, seen superficial to the femoral vessels, and often prominent in the patients with cellulitis whom we often scan in the ER at 2:30 a.m.

533. C. Chronic venous thrombosis.

The structure designated with the cursors is a bright, streaky echo seen frequently in patients with a history of DVT. It represents old, mostly recanalized thrombus that has become organized and dense, creating this bright echo, which will have flow on both sides with color flow.

534. A. Pronounced edema.

All those dark spaces under the skin suggest edema, probably more chronic than acute.

535. A. Cellulitis.

The edema is unlikely to result from either chronic or acute arterial obstruction. Acute DVT and trauma are also unlikely to look like this, as acute edema tends to be more diffuse, without these discrete spaces of collected fluid.

536. D. Brain death.

This characteristic to-and-fro flow pattern has been shown to suggest brain death in cerebral arteries (by TCD), and also in the extracranial ICA, according to work by Tom Rosendahl at Cedars-Sinai Medical Center in Los Angeles.

537. B. Moderately severe (50–80%) stenosis.

By most velocity criteria, a peak systolic velocity >125 cm/sec is compatible with >50% stenosis, while you would want to get the end-diastolic velocity over 100 cm/sec (perhaps well over) to call >80% stenosis. As the caution always goes, you cannot get overly reliant on just the numbers, and you must validate your criteria against angiography, but these numbers are pretty mainstream.

538. C. Immediate angiography.

These repeated TIAs call for action, assuming the patient to be otherwise a reasonable surgical candidate. Since this stenosis falls into a somewhat borderline category (as opposed to being unequivocally >80%), angiography would be the likely next step before going to the OR.

Yes, the NASCET threshold is 70%, and ACAS is 60%, but it does not appear that surgeons are jumping to operate on patients with these thresholds of stenosis at this time.

539. C. Occlusion at the ICA origin.

Here we have a slapping kind of Doppler waveform at the ICA origin—the flow is hitting a brick wall. Note the simultaneous forward and reverse character of the waveform. One must always be extremely cautious, of course, about calling total occlusion; you would first search diligently in the proximal and especially the distal ICA for even a hint of slow flow

getting through a pinhole stenosis. Only then might you call "probable occlusion," noting that duplex is not absolutely reliable at calling these.

540. E. This statement—"The waveform suggests distal occlusion"—is NOT true.

Since there is reasonable diastolic flow, a distal occlusion is unlikely. (Diastolic flow character is determined by distal resistance.) This is another "transitional" vertebral waveform, with late systole being pulled down briefly by a developing abnormal pressure gradient proximally. This is an early stage; examples of later stages appear elsewhere in this book.

541. A. Intraplaque hemorrhage.

One must be careful when suggesting intraplaque hemorrhage, since acoustic shadowing can often create convincing dark areas in a far-wall plaque. However, in this case, the surface of the plaque is readily visible, with a hypoechoic area under it. This image is pretty suggestive of intraplaque hemorrhage. (It does not appear to be creating a severe stenosis, although that is not something best ascertained in the longitudinal image.)

542. E. A and C.

(Okay, too many choices again. Sue me.) This thrombus has the same soft, evenly grainy appearance throughout, compatible with newer thrombus.

543. D. It is a low-resistance waveform.

Because all flow is well above the baseline, this must represent flow to a low-resistance distal vascular bed. It may well be from the brachial artery—okay, it is from the brachial artery—but we can't know that for sure just from this tracing.

544. A. There is something wrong here.

This is a decidedly normal, triphasic arterial waveform. It does not conform to an A/A ratio of 0.56, where you would expect something damped and monophasic.

545. B. Baker's cyst.

It's a fairly large Baker's cyst, a collection of synovial fluid that often causes symptoms similar to those of deep venous thrombosis.

> **Waveforms and Pressures:**
>
> Interpreting this kind of study is widely recognized to be among the most intellectually challenging of vascular lab activities. Some basic principles:

1. Start at the top and look for pressure gradients. A gradient between adjacent cuffs of more than 20–30 mmHg suggests obstruction between the cuffs. (No fair jumping cuffs; they must be adjacent.)

2. High-thigh index should be roughly 1.20, though it can be a bit lower on a slender leg with less cuff artifact. A high-thigh index < 0.80 suggests proximal occlusion. (The indices are given for the low-thigh and calf pressures, but why? There are no criteria for these levels. Just habit, I guess. Ignore these.)

3. Ankle/arm index, of course, is normally equal to or greater than 1.00, but the A/A is mostly helpful when used as a screening tool, not in this full-leg type of study.

4. Use the waveforms to further isolate obstructions. Remember that the waveforms are taken proximal to, between, and distal to the cuffs, not right at the cuff level.
—DR

546. B. Iliac occlusion.

There is something wrong proximal to that monophasic CFA waveform, but it does not affect the left side, where the CFA is multiphasic. So it can't be aortoiliac; it must be confined to the right iliac level. Mainstream pressure-index criteria (see Zwiebel) suggest occlusion when the high-thigh is less than 0.80.

547. E. Within normal limits.

This side is fine: multiphasic waveforms throughout, and all indices > 1.00. (Of course, one would like to perform exercise to see whether the challenge would provoke a pressure drop.)

548. B. Iliac stenosis.

Monophasic but still somewhat sharp CFA waveform, but the problem is again confined to the right iliac level since the left CFA is multiphasic. This time the high-thigh index is reduced but not < 0.80, so we'll call stenosis rather than occlusion.

549. D. Mid posterior tibial stenosis and proximal anterior tibial stenosis.

This is the tricky one. The popliteal waveform is multiphasic, so the problem is probably distal to the popliteal crease. The low-thigh to calf pressure decrease is 38 mmHg to the AT, but only 8 mmHg to the PT. Therefore, there is proximal AT stenosis, while the PT

pressure decrease of 36 mmHg between calf and ankle suggests mid PT stenosis. (Because the decrease is between the cuffs, the problem is between the cuffs.)

550. B. Anterior tibial artery.

From the posteromedial approach, the anterior tibial artery takes off from the popliteal artery (defining the end of that artery) and dives almost directly away from the beam to go (where else?) anteriorly. Newer techs sometimes see a very tempting, prominent branch off the popliteal artery in the popliteal space, but it goes superficial in the field, not deep. Since it is so prominent, they decide it must represent the anterior tibial artery. This is a gastrocnemius (sural) muscular artery, and will move distally to ramify and disappear in the gastrocnemius muscle.

551. C. Demonstrating antegrade flow.

The tibioperoneal trunk is flowing just as it should; this was taken in a student in her twenties. It is blue instead of red because of the direction of flow relative to the color beam (toward). Check the color assignment bar to the left: blue is toward, red is away from the beam.

552. D. Aliasing caused by changing frequency shifts.

The color is indeed aliasing, moving from one color through the brighter hues to the opposite color. The reason is the direction of flow relative to the beam. The flow-to-beam angle at the right of the color box is 70° or even a bit above, making for a rather low frequency shift. The angle in the distal ICA toward the left of the color box is more like 0°, the angle which creates the highest frequency shift. Therefore the colors go brighter and even alias, even though the velocity is probably essentially the same (allowing for a bit of slowing in the carotid bulb). No stenosis here.

Then why does the aliasing occur at the left wall and not the right? Well, the velocities simply aren't the same all the way across the lumen. Flow is a bit faster along the outer portion of a curved segment, just as it is in a meandering river. At least that's my guess.

553. A. Interruption of the color flow due to acoustic shadowing.

This is just more acoustic shadowing, interfering this time not just with the B-mode but also with the color flow. The collateralization answers are fanciful and unlikely.

554. C. The vertical segment is internal carotid artery.

I love to mess with my students with this one. You don't even need to check the color assignment. The superficial branch, ICA, is flowing toward the color beam, and it is blue. The deeper branch is flowing away from the beam, and it is red. That vertical segment is

red, so it must be flowing away from the beam. Therefore, it must represent the continuation of the ICA, which turns to go deep and, on this plane, to overlap with the ECA. (In other words, the vertical segment couldn't be the ECA turning to go up, because it would be toward the beam: blue.)

555. E. A large aneurysm.

This is a big aneurysm, up around 9 to 11 cm.

556. D. This statement—"This is the preferred plane for diameter measurement"—is NOT true of the image presented.

The preferred plane for measuring AAA is longitudinal, not short-axis (see below).

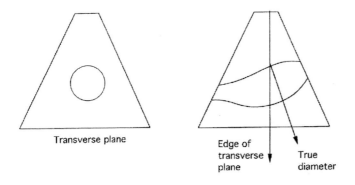

Aneurysms typically have mural thrombus due to stasis against the wall. Aneurysms larger than 5 to 6 cm are usually considered for elective repair, and AAAs are usually infrarenal.

557. E. All of the above.

All are true. The flow going around the tortuosity is swirling in a helical pattern. The reason for those stripes is that the velocities vary somewhat across the lumen. The red flow is what we expect with this color assignment: away from the beam is red. The velocities are somewhat higher on the outer (left) wall, creating an aliased blue display. The white area represents the intermediate zone between the two, as the red assignment moves through white into blue as aliasing occurs.

558. C. This is an artifactual image.

This is the artifact known as "doubling" of an image, caused by a strong reflector—in this case, the pleura near the clavicle. There is only the one subclavian artery, and the deep one is a fake.

559. A. True.

This is a common illustration of how color flow works. The CCA is not quite horizontal all the way across; it has a gentle slope from each side toward the middle. The red display on the left is slightly toward the beam, the blue on the right is slightly away.

560. A. 1, 3, and 5.

Everything is normal. Red flow is away from the beam, so the brachial and ulnar arteries are flowing distally-antegrade. Blue flow is toward the beam, so the radial artery is also flowing distally-antegrade. There is some brachial vein visible above that artery, and some ulnar vein visible above that artery. That blue flow is toward the beam, since that flow is headed cephalad.

561. B. Moderate ICA stenosis.

You can eyeball this, or you can get some calipers and compare the minimal diameter of the proximal ICA to the diameter of the distal unstenosed ICA. Either way, this is moderate stenosis.

562. E. The internal carotid artery.

That's the carotid siphon, where the distal ICA turns anterior, then posterior, just before it bifurcates into middle cerebral and anterior cerebral arteries. The ophthalmic artery does come off the siphon, but the arrow isn't pointing to it.

563. A. Severe SFA stenosis on the right.

You can see some diffuse irregularity along the right superficial femoral artery segment, but there is a focal tight lesion about 3/5 of the way down.

564. E. This statement—"There is high-grade stenosis of the left subclavian artery"—is not true of the angiogram presented.

The left subclavian origin looks okay. All the others are true. Vessel overlap is a common problem with angiography, requiring at least two views from different aspects to get a clear look at the anatomy. (N.B.: All angiograms are shadows created by contrast in the vessels. These shadows are projected onto film, creating these images. Cross your hands over the desk: The shadows overlap.)

565. C. Severe ICA stenosis.

The ICA is on the right in this projection; we know that because the left artery has branches. There's just a small thread of flow at the origin of the ICA. This is pretty severe.

566. C. The superior thyroid artery.

It's the first branch off the ECA, coming off near the origin and heading south.

567. B. Moderate ICA stenosis.

This one is moderate rather than severe, but you can see the wavy protrusion into the lumen of the ICA origin.

568. D. Aortic aneurysm, left iliac occlusion, and right iliac stenosis.

You can just see the right iliac stenosis at lower left of the image. The aneurysm is not severe as yet.

569. C. Right tibioperoneal artery.

Having both right and left images there should help. The right anterior tibial artery is taking its sharp turn to go anterior, but there is no tibioperoneal trunk. Note all the busy collaterals on this side.

570. C. Moderate stenosis of ICA and ECA with probable ulceration.

This is not a particularly severe stenosis of the ICA, but it is rather ugly. Note the shelf-like projection at the proximal end.

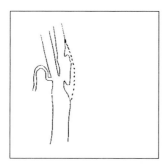

It may take some practice to imagine the original lumen, in order to visualize what the plaque is doing to create these angiographic images. It's a bit of a figure-ground problem. See how the plaque narrows the proximal ICA, then the lumen widens again: This represents a probable crater in the plaque. Then the vessel abruptly narrows again at the distal end of the crater. See the illustration and compare it to the angiogram. You have to draw the dotted line in your mind.

571. B. ICA occlusion and severe ECA stenosis.

The superior thyroid is still there, and some other ECA branches; the ECA itself is a faint shadow, with little contrast making it through. The ICA is gone altogether.

572. B. Occlusion of the left superficial femoral artery with distal reconstitution.

Again, having both right and left helps here. This is the distal end of an SFA occlusion, with reconstitution from the deep femoral artery (coming in from the right side of the image).

573. A. Right renal artery stenosis.

This is a right renal artery stenosis (AP view: patient's right is to your left) just prior to the installation of a stent.

574. C. Abdominal aortic stenosis.

The waviness along the narrowed walls shows moderate diffuse aortic atheroma.

575. A. Vessel overlap, making diagnosis difficult.

This may indeed be a moderate stenosis, but the overlap of the two branches makes it difficult to say for sure. There is something there; note again the wavy intrusion into the lumen, starting in the distal CCA.

PART X

Application for CME Credit

> **Vascular Technology Review**

Vascular Technology Review is a continuing medical educational (CME) activity approved for 12 hours of credit by the Society of Diagnostic Medical Sonographers and may be used by more than one person (see *Note* on page 3).

Who May Apply for CME Credit

This credit may be applied as follows:

* Sonographers and technologists may apply these hours toward the CME requirements of the ARDMS, ARRT, and/or CCI, as well as to the CME requirements of ICAVL for technologists and sonographers in ICAVL-accredited facilities.

* Physicians may apply a certain maximum number of SDMS-approved credit hours toward the CME requirements of the ICAVL for accreditation of diagnostic facilities. (Be sure to confirm current requirements with the pertinent organizations.) Physicians who are registered sonographers or technologists may apply all of these hours toward the CME requirements of the ARDMS, ARRT, and/or CCI. SDMS-approved credit is not applicable toward the AMA Physician's Recognition Award.

If you have any questions whatsoever about CME requirements that affect you, please contact the responsible organization directly for current information. CME requirements can and sometimes do change.

Objectives of this Activity

Upon completion of this educational activity, you will be able to:

1 Describe and identify the anatomy and hemodynamics of the cerebrovascular, venous, peripheral arterial, and abdominal and visceral circulation.
2 Describe how, when, and why imaging and nonimaging techniques are applied to the cerebrovasculature.
3 Describe how, when, and why imaging and nonimaging techniques are applied to the venous system.

4 Describe how, when, and why imaging and nonimaging techniques are applied to the peripheral arterial circulation.
5 Describe how, when, and why imaging and nonimaging techniques are applied to the abdominal and visceral vasculature.
6 Describe the treatment options available to patients with vascular disease.
7 Explain the role and methods of quality assurance and basic patient safety in diagnostic vascular facilities.

How to Obtain CME Credit

1 Read and study the book and complete the interactive exercises it contains.

2 Photocopy and then complete the applicant information page, evaluation questionnaire (you grade us!), and answer sheet.

3 Make copies of the completed forms for your records and then return the originals (i.e., the photocopied forms with your original writing) to the following address for processing:

> **Davies Publishing, Inc.**
> **Attn: CME Coordinator**
> **32 South Raymond Avenue, Suite 4**
> **Pasadena, California 91105-1935**
>
> **Or fax to (626)792-5308**

You may also fax us the applicable pages and pay by credit card. Our fax number is 626-792-5308. You may call us with your credit card, expiration date, and 3- or 4-digit security code or include it with the fax. We grade quizzes within 24 hours of receipt and will email and mail your certificate. Questions? Please call us at 626-792-3046.

4 If more than one person will be applying for credit, be sure to photocopy the applicant information, evaluation form, and CME quiz so that you always have the original on hand for use.

APPLICANT INFORMATION

Name _____   Date of birth _____

Current credentials _____

Home address _____

City/State/Zip _____

Telephone _____   eMail address _____

ARDMS # _____   ARRT # _____   SDMS# _____   CCI# _____

Check enclosed _____

Credit card # _____   Exp date _____   Security code _____

Signature certifying your completion of the activity _____

NOTE

The original purchaser of this CME activity is entitled to submit this CME application for an administrative fee of $39.50. Please enclose a check payable to Davies Publishing Inc. with your application. Others may also submit applications for CME credits by completing the activity as explained above and enclosing an administrative fee of $49.50. The CME administrative fee helps to defray the cost of processing, evaluating, and maintaining a record of your application and the credit you earn. Fees may change without notice. For the current fee, call us at 626.792.3046, e-mail us at **cme@daviespublishing.com**, or write to us at the aforementioned address. We will be happy to help!

Answer sheet, evaluation form, and CME quiz follow . . .

ANSWER SHEET

Circle the correct answer below and return this sheet to Davies Publishing Inc. Passing criterion is 70%. Applicant may not have more than 3 attempts to pass.

1. A B C D E	41. A B C D E	81. A B C D E
2. A B C D E	42. A B C D E	82. A B C D E
3. A B C D E	43. A B C D E	83. A B C D E
4. A B C D E	44. A B C D E	84. A B C D E
5. A B C D E	45. A B C D E	85. A B C D E
6. A B C D E	46. A B C D E	86. A B C D E
7. A B C D E	47. A B C D E	87. A B C D E
8. A B C D E	48. A B C D E	88. A B C D E
9. A B C D E	49. A B C D E	89. A B C D E
10. A B C D E	50. A B C D E	90. A B C D E
11. A B C D E	51. A B C D E	91. A B C D E
12. A B C D E	52. A B C D E	92. A B C D E
13. A B C D E	53. A B C D E	93. A B C D E
14. A B C D E	54. A B C D E	94. A B C D E
15. A B C D E	55. A B C D E	95. A B C D E
16. A B C D E	56. A B C D E	96. A B C D E
17. A B C D E	57. A B C D E	97. A B C D E
18. A B C D E	58. A B C D E	98. A B C D E
19. A B C D E	59. A B C D E	99. A B C D E
20. A B C D E	60. A B C D E	100. A B C D E
21. A B C D E	61. A B C D E	101. A B C D E
22. A B C D E	62. A B C D E	102. A B C D E
23. A B C D E	63. A B C D E	103. A B C D E
24. A B C D E	64. A B C D E	104. A B C D E
25. A B C D E	65. A B C D E	105. A B C D E
26. A B C D E	66. A B C D E	106. A B C D E
27. A B C D E	67. A B C D E	107. A B C D E
28. A B C D E	68. A B C D E	108. A B C D E
29. A B C D E	69. A B C D E	109. A B C D E
30. A B C D E	70. A B C D E	110. A B C D E
31. A B C D E	71. A B C D E	111. A B C D E
32. A B C D E	72. A B C D E	112. A B C D E
33. A B C D E	73. A B C D E	113. A B C D E
34. A B C D E	74. A B C D E	114. A B C D E
35. A B C D E	75. A B C D E	115. A B C D E
36. A B C D E	76. A B C D E	116. A B C D E
37. A B C D E	77. A B C D E	117. A B C D E
38. A B C D E	78. A B C D E	118. A B C D E
39. A B C D E	79. A B C D E	119. A B C D E
40. A B C D E	80. A B C D E	120. A B C D E

Evaluation—You Grade Us!

Please let us know what you think of the *Vascular Technology Review, 4th edition.* Participating in this quality survey is a requirement for CME applicants, and it benefits future readers by ensuring that current readers are satisfied and, if not, that their comments and opinions are heard and taken into account. Your opinions count!

1   Why did you purchase *Vascular Technology Review*? (Circle primary reason.)

   REGISTRY REVIEW   COURSE TEXT   CLINICAL REFERENCE   CME ACTIVITY

2   Have you used *Vascular Technology Review* for other reasons, too? (Circle all that apply.)

   REGISTRY REVIEW   COURSE ACTIVITY   CLINICAL REFERENCE   CME ACTIVITY

3   To what extent did *Vascular Technology Review* meet its stated objectives and your needs? (Circle one.)

   GREATLY   MODERATELY   MINIMALLY   INSIGNIFICANTLY

4   The content of *Vascular Technology Review* was (circle one):

   JUST RIGHT   TOO BASIC   TOO ADVANCED

5   The quality of the questions and explanations was mainly (circle one):

   EXCELLENT   GOOD   FAIR   POOR

6   The manner in which *Vascular Technology Review* presents the material is mainly (circle one):

   EXCELLENT   GOOD   FAIR   POOR

7   If you used this book to prepare for the registry exam, did you also use other materials or take any exam-preparation courses?

   NO   YES (PLEASE SPECIFY WHAT MATERIALS AND COURSES)

   _____
   _____

8   If you used this book for a course, please name the course, the instructor's name, the name of the school or program, and any other textbooks you may have used:

   COURSE/INSTRUCTOR/SCHOOL OR PROGRAM:

   _____

   OTHER TEXTBOOKS:

   _____
   _____

9 What did you like best about *Vascular Technology Review*?

_____
_____
_____

10 What did you like least about *Vascular Technology Review*?

_____
_____
_____

11 If you used *Vascular Technology Review* to prepare for the ARDMS exam in Vascular Technology, did you pass?

YES   NO   HAVEN'T YET TAKEN IT

12 May we quote any of your comments in our catalogs or promotional material?

YES   NO   FURTHER COMMENT . . .

_____
_____
_____
_____
_____
_____
_____
_____
_____
_____
_____
_____
_____
_____

CME QUIZ

Please answer the following questions after you have completed the CME activity. There is one <u>best</u> answer for each question. Circle it on the answer sheet that appears on page 238. Passing criterion is 70%. Applicant may not have more than 3 attempts to pass.

1.   The first branch of the external carotid artery is usually the:

   A. Posterior auricular artery
   B. Inferior thyroid artery
   C. Supraclavicular artery
   D. Superior thyroid artery
   E. Facial artery

2.   The most common variation of the circle of Willis is:

   A. Absence or hypoplasia of one or both of the communicating arteries
   B. Duplication of the posterior communicating arteries
   C. Absence of one of the middle cerebral arteries
   D. Hypoplasia of the proximal segment of one of the anterior cerebral arteries
   E. Duplication of the middle cerebral arteries

3.   What is the most common anatomic variant of the aortic arch?

   A. Duplication of the subclavian arteries
   B. Origin of the right subclavian artery from the aortic arch
   C. Origin of the left vertebral artery from the aortic arch
   D. Origin of the right common carotid artery from the aortic arch
   E. A common origin of the innominate and left common carotid arteries

4.   Which superficial vein receives flow from the three main perforating veins of the distal calf?

   A. Posterior arch vein
   B. Perforator trunk vein
   C. Peroneal vein
   D. Medial malleolar vein
   E. Small saphenous vein

5.   The brachial veins connect the:

   A. Ulnar and radial veins to the subclavian vein
   B. Radial vein to the axillary vein
   C. Ulnar and radial veins to the axillary vein
   D. Radial vein to the subclavian vein
   E. Ulnar vein to the cephalic vein

6.   The vein in the antecubital fossa that connects the cephalic and basilic veins is the:

   A. Ulnar vein
   B. Axillary vein

C. Cephalic vein

D. Median cubital vein

E. Basilic vein

7. The muscular veins of the calf that empty into the popliteal vein behind the knee are the:

A. Perforating veins

B. Gastrocnemius veins

C. Adductor veins

D. Femoral veins

E. Soleal sinuses

8. Which of the following arteries have low-resistance flow character?

A. Internal carotid, postprandial superior mesenteric, and renal arteries

B. External carotid, preprandial superior mesenteric, and renal arteries

C. Internal carotid, preprandial superior mesenteric, and renal arteries

D. Internal carotid and superior mesenteric arteries

E. External carotid, postprandial superior mesenteric, and renal arteries

9. Which of the following is NOT one of the great vessels arising from the aortic arch?

A. Left subclavian artery

B. All arise from the aortic arch

C. Left common carotid artery

D. Innominate artery

E. Right subclavian artery

10. The superior vena cava is formed by the junction of the:

A. Right and left brachiocephalic veins

B. Right and left subclavian veins

C. Innominate and left subclavian veins

D. Inferior vena cava and right innominate vein

E. Innominate and right subclavian veins

11. The artery that supplies the small intestine, right colon, and transverse colon is the:

A. Gastroduodenal

B. Left gastric

C. Superior mesenteric

D. Right gastric

E. Inferior mesenteric

12. Vascular tissue receives its blood supply from the:

A. Tunica vasum

B. Septal capillary networks

C. Osmosis across the intima only

D. Vasa vasorum

E. Media perforators

13. Which of the following statements about atherosclerosis is FALSE?

    A. Atherosclerosis usually develops at bifurcations.
    B. Atherosclerosis is a disease of the red blood cells
    C. Intimal damage/repair may begin in adolescence.
    D. Atherosclerosis is a generalized disease.
    E. Atherosclerosis starts as a breakdown of the intima.

14. What is the next most common source of stroke symptoms after carotid bifurcation disease?

    A. Aortic dissection
    B. Paradoxical embolization from DVT via patent foramen ovale
    C. Spinal stenosis
    D. Subclavian stenosis
    E. Cardiac-source embolization

15. Which statement about subclavian steal is FALSE?

    A. Subclavian steal most commonly occurs on the left side.
    B. It results from severe stenosis or occlusion of the proximal vertebral artery.
    C. All of these statements are false.
    D. Lower blood pressure is seen in the affected arm.
    E. Most patients are asymptomatic.

16. A temporary shading of the vision in one eye is a symptom called:

    A. Dysphasia
    B. Subclavian steal syndrome
    C. Permanent ischemic neurologic event
    D. Reversible ischemic neurologic event
    E. Amaurosis fugax

17. How many new strokes are there each year?

    A. 150,000
    B. 250,000
    C. 500,000
    D. 1,000,000
    E. 2,600,000

18. A TIA resolves within:

    A. 24 hours
    B. 48 hours
    C. 72 hours
    D. 1 week
    E. 10 days

19. "Paresthesia" means:

    A. Tingling sensation
    B. Disturbance of speech
    C. Loss of function of a limb
    D. Weakness
    E. Dizziness

20. Which statement about carotid bruit is FALSE?

    A. A cervical bruit might arise from stenosis of the external carotid artery.
    B. Severe stenosis may cause a bruit.
    C. The presence of a bruit is significant.
    D. The absence of a bruit rules out significant stenosis.
    E. A bruit extending into diastole suggests severe stenosis.

21. When evaluating a patient for cerebrovascular disease, you obtain brachial blood pressures bilaterally because:

    A. It is necessary to know both brachial pressures to rule out the presence of hypoperfusion syndrome.
    B. The systolic components from each arm are averaged to determine the likelihood of cerebrovascular disease.
    C. There is no value in obtaining bilateral brachial pressures if they are not compared to the ankle pressures.
    D. Both brachial blood pressures must be known to determine if hypertension is present.
    E. The brachial blood pressures are compared to see if they are equal.

22. The best duplex image of an arterial wall will be obtained when the beam is at the following angle to the artery walls:

    A. 0°
    B. 60°
    C. 90°
    D. Oblique
    E. Obtuse

23. You are performing a TCD exam. The normal direction of flow in the vertebral artery will be:

    A. Bidirectional
    B. Toward the beam
    C. Away from the beam
    D. Dependent on the cardiac cycle
    E. Undetectable with TCD

24. Which of the following statements about the advantages of continuous-wave Doppler is NOT true?

    A. CW instrumentation is less complex than pulsed-wave Doppler.
    B. Aliasing cannot occur; recording of extremely high frequency shifts is possible.

C. The signal-to-noise ratio is greater than that of pulsed Doppler systems because CW Doppler operates continuously.

D. Continuous-wave Dopplers are less expensive.

E. CW Doppler allows more precise range-gating than pulsed-wave Doppler.

25. A stenosis that reduces the cross-sectional area of an artery by 75% reduces the diameter of that artery by:

   A. 35%
   B. 50%
   C. 60%
   D. 75%
   E. 96%

26. How is the Doppler sample volume usually adjusted?

   A. Big enough to sample flow from a long segment of the artery
   B. Big enough to sample flow from the entire lumen of the artery
   C. Small, to sample flow right against the arterial walls
   D. Small, to sample flow only from center stream
   E. Is not an issue with pulsed-wave Doppler

27. Which of the following color flow adjustments does NOT help to detect slow flow in a possibly occluded internal carotid artery?

   A. Increasing color flow gain
   B. Decreasing color flow PRF
   C. Increasing color flow PRF
   D. Decreasing color flow wall filter
   E. Decreasing beam angle relative to the vessel

28. Which of the following is NOT one of the main collateral pathways in the event of ICA obstruction?

   A. Genicular to arcuate branches
   B. Posterior to anterior
   C. Contralateral hemisphere
   D. ECA branches to ophthalmic branches
   E. All represent major cerebrovascular collateral pathways.

29. Endarterectomy:

   A. Is a relatively recent surgical option
   B. Is used only for carotid stenosis
   C. Is never used for infrarenal arteries
   D. May be used for obstructed lower extremity arteries
   E. Is the treatment of choice for obstructed renal arteries

30. The results of the NASCET trial indicate that the best treatment for carotid stenosis in the symptomatic patient is:

   A. Aspirin for stenosis greater than 70% in diameter

B. Aspirin for stenosis greater than 70% in area

C. Carotid endarterectomy for stenosis greater than 70% in area

D. Carotid endarterectomy for stenosis greater than 70% in diameter

E. Warfarin for stenosis less than 70% in diameter

31. The causes of deep venous thrombosis include:

A. Hypercoagulability

B. Lymphangiitis

C. Extrinsic compression upon deep veins

D. Trauma

E. All except B

32. Virchow's triad includes:

A. Aging, cancer, and bed rest

B. Stasis, increased thrombogenesis, and aging

C. Stasis, aging, and venous injury

D. Stasis, hypercoagulability, and intimal injury

E. Aging, hypercoagulability, and intimal injury

33. A Baker's cyst is a collection of:

A. Red blood cells in a venous sinus

B. Synovial fluid from the knee joint

C. Interstitial fluid along a fascial border

D. Fibrous tissue just beneath the skin

E. White cells and other debris along an infected graft

34. The percentage of untreated calf-vein thrombosis that is thought to propagate to a proximal level (i.e., popliteal or above) is:

A. 3–5%

B. 15–20%

C. 50–60%

D. More than 90%

E. All calf-vein thrombosis propagates at least to the popliteal level

35. Patients suspected of having venous disease may complain of pain that is:

A. Relieved by elevation

B. Not constant

C. Only during the day

D. Not relieved by elevation

E. Mostly felt at night

36. The edema caused by deep venous thrombosis is characterized by:

A. Swelling of the feet

B. Swelling in the ankles and feet

C. Swelling in the ankles, legs, and feet

D. Swelling in the groin

E. Swelling in the ankles and legs but not the feet

37. Lower extremity ulcers are overwhelmingly the result of:

A. Lymphatic disease
B. Arterial disease
C. Venous disease
D. Hyperlipidemia
E. Cardiac disease and chronic right-heart congestion

38. A condition characterized by a severely swollen, blue, cool lower extremity is:

A. Stasis dermatitis
B. Phlegmasia cerulea dolens
C. Cellulitis
D. Phlegmasia alba dolens
E. Lymphedema

39. A common physical finding in pulmonary embolism is:

A. Tachypnea
B. Bradycardia
C. Thrombocytopenia
D. Bradypenia
E. Apnea

40. During a duplex venous exam, which of the following findings is the least likely to be associated with acute deep venous thrombosis?

A. Homogeneous intraluminal echoes
B. Continuous venous flow
C. Stationary echoes within the vein
D. Enlarged incompressible vein
E. Venous reflux

41. The Valsalva maneuver:

A. Affects arterial, not venous, flow
B. Slows down or stops venous flow everywhere in the body
C. Decreases pressure in the thoracic cavity, increases pressure in the abdominal cavity
D. Increases venous flow everywhere in the body
E. Increases pressure in the thoracic cavity, decreases pressure in the abdominal cavity

42. The duplex venous imaging findings that suggest acute rather than chronic deep vein thrombosis include all EXCEPT:

A. Presence of a "tail" suggesting poor adherence to wall
B. Distended vein
C. Dark intraluminal echoes
D. Slightly compressible (spongy) character to thrombus

E. Bright intraluminal echoes

43. Pulsatility of lower extremity venous Doppler signals would be associated with:

   A. CVA
   B. Acute arterial occlusion
   C. Severe superficial vein valvular insufficiency
   D. Congestive heart failure
   E. Deep vein thrombosis

44. Descending venography is performed to diagnose:

   A. Valvular insufficiency
   B. Superficial venous thrombosis
   C. Popliteal venous thrombosis
   D. Femoral venous thrombosis
   E. Inferior vena cava valvular insufficiency

45. The current standard of treatment for deep venous thrombosis consists of placing the patient on the following medication for 3 or more months following the initial dose of heparin:

   A. Sodium warfarin
   B. Urokinase
   C. Tissue plasminogen activator
   D. Vitamin K
   E. Streptokinase

46. More than 90% of infrarenal abdominal aneurysms are of:

   A. Syphilitic origin
   B. Infectious origin
   C. Anastomotic origin
   D. Degenerative origin
   E. Traumatic origin

47. Aneurysms are most often caused by:

   A. Trauma
   B. Systemic infection
   C. Pregnancy
   D. Bifurcated laminar flow
   E. Congenital arterial wall weakness

48. The most common site of atherosclerosis in the lower extremity is:

   A. The arterial segment at the iliac bifurcation
   B. The arterial segment beginning at the popliteal artery
   C. The arterial segment beginning in Hunter's canal
   D. The arterial segment at the popliteal trifurcations
   E. The proximal tibial vessels

49. Which of the following is NOT a risk factor in peripheral arterial occlusive disease?

    A. Hypolipidemia
    B. Hyperlipidemia
    C. Hypertension
    D. Diabetes
    E. Smoking

50. *Cyanosis* is:

    A. Thickening of toenails due to chronic ischemia
    B. Red color of tissue due to hyperemia
    C. Pale skin due to ischemia
    D. Blue color of tissue due to ischemia
    E. Loss of hair growth due to chronic ischemia

51. You are examining a patient who developed a pulsatile mass in the groin after undergoing cardiac catheterization. This mass is most likely a(n):

    A. Femoral artery aneurysm
    B. Hematoma
    C. Pseudoaneurysm of the femoral artery
    D. False aneurysm of the femoral vein
    E. Arteriovenous fistula

52. A vibration noted while palpating pulses is a:

    A. Thrill
    B. Bruit
    C. Scintillation
    D. Pulse
    E. Buzz

53. Delayed return of the capillary blush after pressure on the pulp of the digit is a sign of:

    A. Hypercholesterolemia
    B. Advanced ischemia
    C. Venous occlusive disease
    D. Hyperlipidemia
    E. Thoracic outlet syndrome

54. Unilateral claudication in the calf and foot of a young individual suggests:

    A. Arteriosclerosis
    B. Anterior tibial compartment syndrome
    C. "Restless" leg syndrome
    D. Lumbar disc disease
    E. Popliteal artery entrapment

55. The pulsatility index is calculated as follows:

    A. Peak systolic velocity minus end diastolic velocity divided by systolic velocity.
    B. Peak systolic to peak end diastolic velocity divided by mean velocity.
    C. Peak systolic velocity minus mean velocity divided by systolic velocity.
    D. Peak systolic velocity divided by end diastolic velocity.
    E. Peak systolic velocity at the internal carotid artery divided by peak systolic velocity at the common carotid artery.

56. The two flow characteristics that define arterial stenosis anywhere in the body include focal acceleration of velocities and:

    A. Decreased diastolic flow
    B. Decreased resistance proximally
    C. Increased flow reversal
    D. Increased pulsatility distally
    E. Distal turbulence

57. This CW Doppler waveform from a popliteal artery:

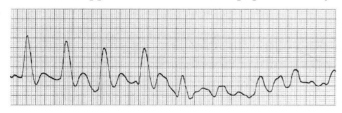

    A. Suggests interference from venous flow
    B. Is severely abnormal in character
    C. Is a normal arterial waveform
    D. Is monophasic
    E. Suggests femoral artery occlusion

58. Your patient has the following segmental pressure readings:

Rt. brachial: 144 mmHg	Lt. Brachial: 140
Rt. high thigh: 110	Lt. high thigh: 164

    These findings could result from all EXCEPT:

    A. Right common femoral obstruction
    B. Right common iliac obstruction
    C. Right external iliac obstruction
    D. Aortoiliac obstruction
    E. Right proximal superficial femoral obstruction

59. Distal to an aortoiliac occlusion, the common femoral artery signal is typically:

    A. High-pitched
    B. Biphasic
    C. Multiphasic
    D. Low-pitched and monophasic

E. Impossible to distinguish from a pulsatile venous signal

60. Audible Doppler venous signals typically are low-frequency and vary with respiration, whereas normal arterial signals in the legs and arms are:

    A. Low-frequency yet pulsatile
    B. Multiphasic and vary with respiration
    C. Relatively high-frequency and nonpulsatile
    D. Relatively high-frequency with pulsatile components
    E. Multiphasic and phasic with respiration

61. You are examining a patient who wakes up at night with pain in the foot and has to drop the foot by the side of the bed. This patient's ankle/arm systolic pressure ratio will most likely be:

    A. Greater than 1.00
    B. Between 0.80 and 1.00
    C. Between 0.50 and 0.80
    D. Less than 0.50
    E. Not measurable

62. A damped Doppler velocity waveform of the subclavian artery isolates a significant lesion:

    A. At or distal to the brachial artery
    B. Near the origin of the subclavian artery
    C. Proximal to the point of insonation
    D. To the vertebral artery
    E. To the innominate artery

63. When calculating ankle/brachial systolic pressure ratios, which of the following arm pressures is commonly selected as the denominator?

    A. The lower of the right or left arm pressures
    B. The higher of the right or left arm pressures
    C. The left arm pressure
    D. The right arm pressure
    E. Random selection of the right or left arm pressure

64. On angiography, the appearance of a "string of beads" is typical of:

    A. Polyarteritis nodosa
    B. Fibromuscular dysplasia
    C. Takayasu's arteritis
    D. Raynaud's syndrome
    E. Diabetes mellitus

65. Which of these drugs is commonly used to treat claudication?

    A. Dipiridamole
    B. Heparin
    C. Coumadin

D. Aspirin

E. Pletal

66. For acute arterial thrombosis, the most effective lytic treatment is:

A. tPA

B. Heparin

C. Sodium warfarin

D. Vasopressors

E. Inotropic agents

67. Atherosclerotic disease of the renal artery is most commonly found in the following location:

A. Proximal

B. Mid

C. Distal

D. Intrarenal

E. The disease strikes all of these sites with about the same frequency.

68. The Budd-Chiari syndrome is a cause of portal hypertension resulting from:

A. A liver tumor

B. Inferior mesenteric vein thrombus

C. Hepatic vein obstruction

D. Superior vena cava thrombus

E. Hepatic artery stenosis

69. The patient with advanced chronic mesenteric ischemia is most likely to be:

A. Obese

B. Malnourished

C. In atrial fibrillation

D. Hyperactive

E. Free of discernable symptoms

70. Which of the following conditions is a common manifestation of portal hypertension?

A. Claudication

B. Homonymous hemianopia

C. Vasculogenic impotence

D. Bleeding esophageal varices

E. Clubbing of digits

71. Which of the following abdominal arteries normally demonstrates higher diastolic flow postprandially?

A. Superior mesenteric

B. Common hepatic

C. Splenic

D. Renal

E. Celiac axis

72. Pulsatility of the hepatic vein Doppler signal may suggest:

    A. Tricuspid regurgitation
    B. Hepatic metastases
    C. Hepatic artery thrombosis
    D. Hepatic infarction
    E. Normal flow

73. Normal flow in the hepatic vein is:

    A. Retrograde
    B. Hepatopetal
    C. Triphasic
    D. Not detectable with duplex
    E. Bidirectional

74. A normal penile/brachial systolic pressure ratio is:

    A. > 3.5:1
    B. > 0.45
    C. > 1.3
    D. > 0.5
    E. > 0.75

75. An abnormal flow rate for a radial artery/cephalic vein dialysis fistula is:

    A. 200 to 400 ml/min
    B. 400 to 900 ml/min
    C. 1000 to 1500 ml/min
    D. Greater than 1500 ml/min
    E. Less than 200 ml/min

76. Temporal arteritis is commonly characterized by:

    A. Dissection
    B. Aneurysm
    C. Tortuosity
    D. Intimal thickening
    E. Ectasia

77. The probability that a positive noninvasive test reveals actual disease (as diagnosed by the gold-standard test) is called:

    A. Specificity
    B. Sensitivity
    C. Accuracy
    D. Negative predictive value
    E. Positive predictive value

78. Correlating a noninvasive test to its gold standard, you calculate a sensitivity of 93%. You know that the specificity must be:

    A. Greater than the sensitivity.
    B. Less than the sensitivity.
    C. Equal to the sensitivity.
    D. Within 10 to 15% of the sensitivity.
    E. A value from 0 to 100%.

79. Which condition is associated with compression of subclavian artery and brachial plexus by the cervical rib?

    A. Thoracic outlet syndrome
    B. Cervical spine disease
    C. Subclavian steal syndrome
    D. Causalgia
    E. Vertebral stenosis

80. Normally a Doppler signal from the subclavian vein is expected to be:

    A. Pulsatile
    B. Triphasic
    C. Absent in older patients
    D. Nonspontaneous except in warm patients
    E. Retrograde

81. Of the following symptoms, which can be attributed to the vertebrobasilar system?

    A. Vertigo
    B. Aphasia
    C. Unilateral paresis
    D. Amaurosis fugax
    E. Right anterior hemisphere TIA

82. A normal hepatic vein spectral waveform is:

    A. Unidirectional
    B. Triphasic
    C. Continuous
    D. Bidirectional
    E. A and C

83. Which of the following statements about subclavian steal is accurate?

    A. Mainly in females
    B. Mainly in young, male smokers
    C. More often on the right side
    D. Equally often on both sides
    E. More often on the left side

84. What two arteries does the axillary artery connect?

    A. Brachial artery to the radial artery
    B. Radial to the ulnar artery
    C. Ulnar to the brachial artery
    D. Brachial artery to the subclavian artery
    E. Radial to the subclavian artery

85. In the lower extremity venous exam it is usually most difficult to bring about vein-wall coaptation with probe compression in:

    A. The saphenofemoral junction
    B. The mid calf
    C. The popliteal space
    D. The distal thigh
    E. The mid thigh

86. The tiny intrarenal branches that arise from the interlobar arteries at right angles and course above the renal pyramids are the:

    A. Segmental arteries
    B. Interlobular arteries
    C. Intralobular arteries
    D. Capsular arteries
    E. Arcuate arteries

87. What is the most common medical treatment of acute ischemic stroke?

    A. Dipyridamole
    B. rtPA
    C. Dextran
    D. Heparin
    E. Aspirin

88. Where is Boyd's perforating vein located?

    A. Near the knee
    B. In the distal thigh
    C. On the dorsum of the foot
    D. In the proximal thigh
    E. In the lower calf

89. "TIA" is an abbreviation for?

    A. Temporary ischemic attack
    B. Terminal internal artery
    C. Transient internal artery
    D. Temporary internal attack
    E. Transient ischemic attack

90. Which of the following devices, utilized in a standard fashion, can NOT measure ankle pressures?

   A. B-mode ultrasound
   B. Doppler ultrasound
   C. Strain-gauge plethysmography
   D. Air plethysmography
   E. Photocell plethysmography

91. *RIND*, also called *stroke with recovery*, is:

   A. A neurologic deficit that does not resolve.
   B. A neurologic ischemic deficit that resolves completely after 24 hours.
   C. A neurologic deficit that waxes and wanes.
   D. A reversible ischemic neurologic deficit that completely resolves within 24 hours.
   E. An irreversible neurologic deficit.

92. In a normal individual, the ankle-pressure response to reactive hyperemia is:

   A. A transient increase of approximately 50%
   B. A transient decrease of approximately 20%
   C. A quick, transient drop of greater than 50%
   D. A gradual decrease of approximately 50%
   E. A gradual increase of approximately 50%

93. Name a useful landmark for locating the renal arteries:

   A. Common hepatic artery
   B. Right renal vein
   C. Celiac axis
   D. Superior mesenteric artery
   E. Inferior mesenteric artery

94. The circle of Willis receives its blood supply from which combination of arteries?

   A. Internal and external carotid arteries
   B. Right and left vertebral arteries
   C. Carotid and vertebral arteries
   D. Subclavian and vertebral arteries
   E. Posterior cerebral artery and basilar artery

95. Venules consist of these layers:

   A. Tunica media and tunica adventitia
   B. Tunica media and tunica intima
   C. Tunica adventitia and tunica media
   D. Tunica adventitia and tunica intima
   E. Tunica adventitia, tunica media, and tunica intima

96. For assessing the carotid arteries, which imaging transducer frequency would be appropriate?

    A. 0.3 MHz
    B. 2.5 MHz
    C. 5 MHz
    D. 10 MHz
    E. C and D

97. It is useful to assess the patency of the palmar arch:

    A. When evaluating a patient with suspected subclavian steal
    B. Before placement of an arteriovenous arm shunt
    C. To evaluate blood flow to the digital arteries
    D. A and B
    E. B and C

98. Which of the following vessels and structures is NOT a part of the penis?

    A. Deep artery of the penis
    B. Corpus spongiosum
    C. Inferior vesicle artery
    D. Dorsal artery of the penis
    E. Dorsal vein

99. On duplex exam, all of the following are indications of a totally occluded internal carotid artery EXCEPT:

    A. No Doppler or color flow obtainable within ICA lumen
    B. ICA lumen filled with heterogeneous echoes
    C. Absence of diastolic flow in CCA spectral display
    D. "Drumbeat" or "slapping" Doppler signal at ICA origin
    E. Greatly increased end-diastolic velocities in CCA spectral display

100. Back, abdominal, or flank pain is associated with which vascular disease?

    A. Intracranial arterial disease
    B. Renal artery stenosis
    C. Iliofemoral occlusive disease
    D. Abdominal aortic aneurysm
    E. Superior mesenteric stenosis

101. What is the first major arterial branch of the aorta?

    A. The right subclavian artery
    B. The left subclavian artery
    C. The left common carotid artery
    D. The right common carotid artery
    E. The innominate artery

102. Which of the following conditions would NOT produce symptoms of chronic venous insufficiency?

    A. Gastrocnemius muscular thrombosis
    B. Calf-vein thrombosis
    C. Superficial insufficiency
    D. Popliteal vein thrombosis
    E. Iliac vein thrombosis

103. How is the ankle/arm index calculated?

    A. By dividing the ankle pressure by the average of the two brachial pressures
    B. By dividing the lower of the two brachial pressures by ankle pressure
    C. By dividing the ankle pressure by the lower brachial pressure
    D. By dividing the higher of the two brachial pressures by ankle pressure
    E. By dividing the ankle pressure by the higher brachial pressure

104. Your patient begins to fall while getting off the examination table. You should:

    A. Catch him under the arms.
    B. Guide the fall, protecting his head.
    C. Catch him around the waist.
    D. Start filling out the incident report.
    E. Let him fall, since you may just hurt him worse by interfering.

105. What is the "tunica intima"?

    A. Longitudinal muscle fibers
    B. Transverse arterial muscle fibers
    C. The inner lining of the arterial wall
    D. The middle layer of the arterial wall
    E. The outer lining of the arterial wall

106. Your TCD exam demonstrates normal direction of flow in the middle cerebral artery. The flow is:

    A. Dependent on the cardiac cycle
    B. Toward the beam
    C. Bidirectional
    D. Away from the beam
    E. Not detectable with TCD

107. The structure forming the prominence of the larynx is the:

    A. Greater cornu
    B. Cricoid cartilage
    C. Thyroid gland
    D. Thyroid cartilage
    E. Hyoid bone

108. What is the most prevalent type of stroke?

    A. Septic embolic
    B. Hemorrhagic
    C. Ischemic
    D. Aneurysmal
    E. Venous thrombotic

109. Of the following, which is least likely to contribute to DVT?

    A. Pregnancy and delivery
    B. Previous DVT
    C. Diabetes
    D. Pelvic mass
    E. Hip replacement surgery

110. A patient presents with stroke symptoms in the E.R. The initial diagnostic exam of choice would likely be:

    A. Carotid duplex
    B. MRI
    C. Radionucleotide study
    D. CT
    E. Cerebral angiography

111. What is the most common cause of portal hypertension in the United States?

    A. Cirrhosis
    B. Hepatic carcinoma
    C. Schistosomiasis
    D. Hypertension
    E. Hyperlipidemia

112. The brachial veins form the axillary vein when they join the:

    A. Basilic vein
    B. Subclavian vein
    C. Cephalic vein
    D. Innominate vein
    E. Ulnar vein

113. A complication of plaque ulceration is:

    A. Thrombosis
    B. Embolization
    C. Intraplaque hemorrhage
    D. All of the above
    E. None of the above

114. A patient with pulmonary embolism may present with any of the following symptoms EXCEPT:

    A. Tachypnea
    B. Dyspnea
    C. Positive lower extremity venous ultrasound
    D. Pleural effusion
    E. Chest pain

115. The junction of which two veins forms the superior vena cava?

    A. Right and left brachiocephalic veins
    B. Right and left subclavian veins
    C. Inferior vena cava and right innominate vein
    D. Innominate and left subclavian veins
    E. Innominate and right subclavian veins

116. Takayasu's arteritis most commonly afflicts:

    A. Young men
    B. Young women
    C. Middle-aged men
    D. Elderly men
    E. Elderly women

117. The condition that is least likely to cause a bruit in the neck is:

    A. Critical preocclusive stenosis of the internal carotid artery
    B. Hyperdynamic carotid flows
    C. Cardiac valvular disease
    D. Severe stenosis of the external carotid artery
    E. Severe stenosis of the internal carotid artery

118. What is the term for the smallest vessels in the body:

    A. Adventitias
    B. Capillaries
    C. Venules
    D. Arterioles
    E. Intimas

119. Atherosclerosis in the cerebrovascular system usually develops in the:

    A. Intracranial internal carotid artery
    B. Proximal common carotid artery
    C. Origin of internal carotid artery
    D. Innominate artery
    E. Left subclavian artery

120. What is considered to be the optimal Doppler beam angle for standardization of duplex carotid studies at most vascular labs?

    A. Any angle greater than 60°
    B. 60°
    C. 40–45°
    D. 20–40°
    E. 0°

PART XI

Exam Outline

The American Registry of Diagnostic Medical Sonographers publishes its exam outlines and other important information on its website (www.ARDMS.org). Visit the site for complete information about applying for and taking the registry examinations. The outline for each exam indicates the approximate percentage of the exam that a particular topic represents. This information is important because is indicates the relative importance of each topic and allows you to study more effectively. For example, the topic of protocols represents 33% of the Vascular Technology exam, whereas patient care represents 4%.

The complete outline for the Vascular Technology specialty examination appears below.

I.   Anatomy & Physiology (20%)

    A. Cerebrovascular

        1. Cerebrovascular normal anatomy

        2. Cerebrovascular hemodynamics

    B. Venous

        1. Venous normal anatomy

        2. Venous hemodynamics

    C. Peripheral Arterial

        1. Peripheral arterial normal anatomy

        2. Peripheral arterial hemodynamics

    D. Abdominal/Visceral

        1. Abdominal/visceral normal anatomy

        2. Abdominal/visceral hemodynamics

II. Pathology (19%)

    A. Cerebrovascular

        1. Cerebrovascular abnormal perfusion and physiology

        2. Cerebrovascular postoperative (surgically corrected) anatomy

    B. Venous

        1. Venous abnormal perfusion and physiology

        2. Venous postoperative (surgically corrected) anatomy

    C. Peripheral Arterial

        1. Peripheral arterial abnormal perfusion and physiology

        2. Peripheral arterial postoperative (surgically corrected) anatomy

    D. Abdominal/Visceral

        1. Abdominal/visceral abnormal perfusion and physiology

        2. Abdominal/visceral postoperative (surgically corrected) anatomy

III. Patient Care (4%)

    A. Communication

IV. Integration of Data (10%)

    A. Cerebrovascular

        1. Cerebrovascular incorporate outside data (clinical assessment, health & physical [H&P], lab values, risk factors)

        2. Cerebrovascular interpretation (differential diagnosis)

    B. Venous

        1. Venous incorporate outside data (clinical assessment, health & physical [H&P], lab values, risk factors)

        2. Venous interpretation (differential diagnosis)

    C. Peripheral Arterial

        1. Peripheral arterial incorporate outside data (clinical assessment, health & physical [H&P], lab values, risk factors)

        2. Peripheral arterial interpretation (differential diagnosis)

    D. Abdominal/Visceral

        1. Abdominal/visceral incorporate outside data (clinical assessment, health & physical [H&P], lab values, risk factors)

        2. Abdominal/visceral interpretation (differential diagnosis)

V. Protocols (33%)

    A. Cerebrovascular

        1. Cerebrovascular clinical standards and guidelines

        2. Cerebrovascular measurement techniques

    B. Venous

1. Venous clinical standards and guidelines

2. Venous measurement techniques

3. Venous non-sonographic techniques

C. Peripheral Arterial

1. Peripheral arterial clinical standards and guidelines

2. Peripheral arterial measurement techniques

3. Peripheral arterial non-sonographic techniques

D. Abdominal/Visceral

1. Abdominal/visceral clinical standards and guidelines

2. Abdominal/visceral measurement techniques

E. Physics and Instrumentation (5%)

1. Artifacts

2. Imaging instruments

3. Quality assurance/statistics

VI. Treatment (7%)

A. Cerebrovascular

1. Cerebrovascular intraoperative procedures

B. Venous

1. Venous intraoperative procedures

C. Peripheral arterial

1. Peripheral arterial intraoperative procedures

2. Peripheral arterial sonographer role in procedures

D. Abdominal/Visceral

1. Abdominal/visceral intraoperative procedures

VII. Other (2%)

A. Traumatic injury

B. Miscellaneous conditions/tests

PART XII

Bibliography

PRIMARY REFERENCES

Belanger A: *Vascular Anatomy and Physiology*. Pasadena, CA, Davies Publishing, 1999.

Bergan J (ed): *The Vein Book*. St. Louis, Elsevier Academic Press, 2007.

Bernstein EF: *Vascular Diagnosis*, 4th edition. St. Louis, Mosby, 1993.

Pellerito JS, Polak JF: *Introduction to Vascular Ultrasonography*, 6th edition. Philadelphia, Elsevier Saunders, 2012.

Ridgway DP: *Introduction to Vascular Scanning: A Guide for the Complete Beginner*, 4th edition. Pasadena, CA, Davies Publishing, 2014.

Rumwell CB, McPharlin M: *Vascular Technology: An Illustrated Review*, 5th edition. Pasadena, CA, Davies Publishing, 2015.

Rutherford RB: *Vascular Surgery*, 5th edition. Philadelphia, Saunders, 2000.

Zwiebel WJ: *Introduction to Vascular Ultrasonography*, 5th edition. Philadelphia, Saunders, 2005.

FURTHER READING

Hershey FA, Barnes RW, Sumner DE: *Noninvasive Diagnosis of Vascular Disease*. Pasadena, CA, Davies Publishing, 1983.

Kremkau FW: *Sonography: Principles and Instruments*, 8th edition. St. Louis, Elsevier Saunders, 2011.

Kremkau FW: *Diagnostic Ultrasound: Principles and Instruments*, 7th edition. Philadelphia, Saunders, 2006.
Owen CA, Strandness DE Jr: *ScoreCards for Vascular Technology*. Pasadena, CA, Davies Publishing, 2009.

Salles-Cunha SX, Andros GW: *Atlas of Duplex Ultrasonography*. Pasadena, CA, Davies Publishing, 1992.